WRITERS REPUBLIC

WRITERS REPUBLIC L.L.C.
515 Summit Ave. Unit R1
Union City, NJ 07087, USA

Website: *www.writersrepublic.com*
Hotline: *1-877-656-6838*
Email: *info@writersrepublic.com*

Ordering Information:
Quantity sales. Special discounts are available on quantity purchases by corporations, associations, and others. For details, contact the publisher at the address above.

Library of Congress Control Number: 2023905863
ISBN-13:   978-1-64620-176-1   [Paperback Edition]
                  979-8-88810-915-1   [Hardback Edition]
                  978-1-64620-177-8   [Digital Edition]

Rev. date: 03/23/2023

ABOUT THE BOOK

The Veterinary Technician's Guide to Emergency and Critical Care Volume I is a comprehensive manual to have on your bookshelf and in your pocket at all times with articles in Small Animal Critical Care Veterinary Medicine, useful tables and charts, tips and tricks, pharmacology, drug reconstitution, dilution, and calculation, various blood testing procedures, how to monitor and respond to the critical patient in a variety of situations and scenarios, and so much more!

This guide contains the constant rate infusion calculations for the most utilized drugs in E.C.C. and shows you the step-by-step instructions for each of the equations in linear algebra, and not dimensional analysis. This guide is not for the layperson, but it does explain difficult concepts thoroughly for those well-versed in Veterinary Medicine and this specialty.

This guide is perfect for Veterinary Technicians, Veterinary Students, Technician Students, and even Doctors looking to have information easily accessible for making decisions quickly when patient care is at stake.

This book is dedicated
to my family.
Thank you for your
unwavering support and love.

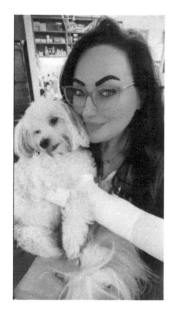
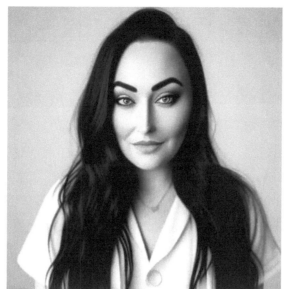
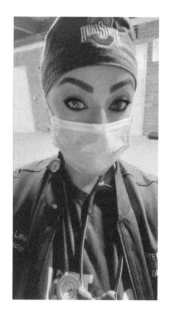

ABOUT THE AUTHOR

Kristin Lake is an Emergency and Critical Care Veterinary Technician that has been working in the field since 2003 when she graduated high school and started in General Practice. She then moved into specialties like Medical Oncology, Large Animal and Equine Medicine, Mobile Veterinary Medicine, Shelter Animal Medicine, Emergency and Critical Care Medicine for Domestic and Exotic Animals including Anesthesia. She received her Bachelor of Science degree from the University of Maryland in 2014 as a Social Science major and Biology minor with concentrations in Medical Sociology, Global Public Health, Epidemiology, Infectious Disease, Veterinary Public Health, Biosecurity and much more. She was a Board Member for her local Animal Matters Hearing Board and elected to two consecutive terms by the Charles County, MD Commissioners Office to oversee, hear, and rule on all civil complaints and Animal Control citations issued to citizens, as well as all non-felony animal cruelty cases occurring in Charles County, MD. She participates in volunteer work with Veterinary Technician students at Appalachian State University and helps to teach Veterinary Technicians and Assistants medical math through social media. In 2023 her first book was released entitled, 'The Veterinary Technician's Guide to Emergency and Critical Care' and she started VetMedMath.com to tutor veterinary professionals in medical math. She hopes to begin lecturing on a variety of topics at veterinary conventions by 2024.

TABLE OF CONTENTS

CHAPTER 1:   PAGE 6
NORMAL VITALS &
MAINTENANCE FLUID RATES

CHAPTER 2:   PAGE 15
BOLUS RATES, SHOCK BOLUSES
& INTRAVENOUS FLUID
RESUSCITATION

CHAPTER 3:   PAGE 29
DRUG CONCENTRATIONS

CHAPTER 4:   PAGE 33
ALGEBRA REVIEW

CHAPTER 5:   PAGE 36
TOXICOLOGY

CHAPTER 6:   PAGE 44
RECOVER PROTOCOL
INTRATRACHEAL DRUG
ADMINISTRATION & ADVANCED
VENOUS ACCESS

CHAPTER 7:   PAGE 51
CONSTANT RATE INFUSIONS

CHAPTER 8:   PAGE 87
IV FLUID ADDITIVES

CHAPTER 9:   PAGE 102
VESICANTS & IRRITANTS

CHAPTER 10:   PAGE 107
INSULIN CRI, IV DRUG
ADMINISTRATION, DEXDOMITOR
CRI & PROPOFOL CRI

CHAPTER 11:   PAGE 117
20% MANNITOL

CHAPTER 12:   PAGE 120
URINARY OUTPUT, SENSIBLE &
INSENSIBLE LOSSES

TABLE OF CONTENTS

CHAPTER 13:   PAGE 123
HOW TO PLACE A MODIFIED
ROBERT JONES BANDAGE

CHAPTER 14:   PAGE 126
VENOMVET SNAKE BITE
ENVENOMATION PROTOCOL

CHAPTER 15:   PAGE 175
ANESTHESIA SHEET

CHAPTER 16:   PAGE 180
TIPS & TRICKS FROM
VETERINARY PROFESSIONALS

CHAPTER 17:   PAGE 184
CAPNOGRAPHY

CHAPTER 18:   PAGE 187
EMERGENCY MEDICINE AND
HOW TO THRIVE IN AN
UKNOWN ENVIRONMENT

CHAPTER 19:   PAGE 191
CITATIONS

CHAPTER 1:
NORMAL VITALS & MAINTENANCE FLUID RATES

NORMAL RATES FOR VITALS

HR

DOGS	60 – 140 BPM	
CATS	160 – 240 BPM	

RR

DOGS	12 – 40 RPM	
CATS	16 – 40 RPM	

TEMP

DOGS	100.5 ° – 102.5 °	
CATS	100.5 ° – 102.5 °	

Pro Tip

*FOR DOGS, CALCULATE HR AND RR BY COUNTING HOW MANY BEATS OR RESPIRATIONS YOU HEAR IN 15 SECONDS THEN MULTIPLY BY 4.

*YOU CAN ALSO COUNT HOW MANY BEATS OR RESPIRATIONS YOU HEAR IN 10 SECONDS AND MULTIPLY BY 6.

*FOR CATS: CALCULATE HR BY COUNTING HOW MANY BEATS YOU HEAR IN 5 SECONDS THEN MULTIPLY BY 12.

MAINTENANCE FLUID RATES

Dehydration can be corrected over 24 to 48 hours. Once the deficit has been determined, the total volume can be divided by the number of hours over which the dehydration is to be corrected to obtain a mL/h rate.

Maintenance fluid needs are based on both sensible and insensible losses. These can be estimated as 40-60 ml/kg/day or **2-3 ml/kg per hour** in adults (pediatric patients require slightly higher rates).

As an example, the daily fluid needs of a 5-kg patient that is estimated to be 6% dehydrated (to be corrected over 24 hours) and has estimated ongoing losses of 1 mL/kg per hour can be calculated as follows:

- Dehydration deficit: 5 kg × 0.06 = 0.3 L × 1000 = 300 mL to be corrected over 24 hours (300 mL/24 hr) = 12.5 mL/hr
- Maintenance rate: 2 mL/kg/hr × 5 kg = 10 mL/hr
- Ongoing losses: 1 mL/kg/hr × 5 kg = 5 mL/hr
- Total rate (dehydration + maintenance + losses): 12.5 + 10 + 5 = 27.5 mL/hr

ESTIMATED DEHYDRATION	PHYSICAL EXAMINATION FINDINGS
<5%	Not detectable
5% – 6%	Tacky mucous membranes
6% – 8%	Decreased skin turgor Dry mucous membranes
8% – 10%	Retracted globes within orbits
10% – 12%	Persistent skin tent Dull corneas Evidence of hypovolemia
>12%	Hypovolemic shock Death

MUIR WW, DIBARTOLA SP. FLUID THERAPY. IN: KIRK RW. ED. *CURRENT VETERINARY THERAPY VIII*. PHILADELPHIA: WB SAUNDERS; 1983:33.

TABLE 1 (Lyons and Waddell, 2019)

For the first 24 hours of hospitalization, correct 80% of the dehydration deficit. If calculating fluids over 12 hours, do not calculate the 80% correction of the dehydration deficit.

EXAMPLE

CANINE
Order: 1xM = 60 ML/KG/DAY
Weight: 12KG
Dehydration Deficit: 5% Dehydrated
Time: 24 Hours

Maintenance Rate:

60 ML/~~KG~~/DAY x 12 ~~KG~~ = 720 ML/DAY
720 ML/~~DAY~~ / 24 HR/~~DAY~~ = 30 ML/HR

Dehydration Deficit:

12 ~~KG~~ x 0.05 L/~~KG~~ (5% in decimal form) = 0.6 L (L= Liters)
0.6 ~~L~~ x 1000 ML/~~L~~ = 600 ML
600 ML x 0.8 (80% in decimal form) = 480 ML
480 ML / 24 HR = 20 ML/HR

+/- Estimated Ongoing Losses:

1 ML/~~KG~~/HR x 12 ~~KG~~ = 12 ML/HR

CALCULATION OF MAINTENANCE RATE, DEHYDRATION DEFICIT AND ESTIMATED ONGOING LOSSES:

30 ML/HR (MAINTENANCE) + 20 ML/HR (DEHYDRATION DEFICIT) + 12 ML/HR (ESTIMATED ONGOING LOSSES) = 62 ML/HR

CALCULATION WITHOUT ESTIMATED ONGOING LOSSES:

30 ML/HR (MAINTENANCE) + 20 ML/HR (DEHYDRATION DEFICIT) = 50 ML/HR

EXAMPLE

FELINE
Order: 1xM = 40 ML/KG/DAY
Weight: 5KG
Dehydration Deficit: 5% Dehydrated
Time: 12 Hours

Maintenance Rate:

40 ML/~~KG~~/DAY x 5 ~~KG~~ = 200 ML/DAY
200 ML/~~DAY~~ / 12 HR/~~DAY~~ = 16.6 ML/HR

Dehydration Deficit:

5 ~~KG~~ x 0.05 L/~~KG~~ (5% in decimal form) = 0.25 L
0.25 ~~L~~ x 1000 ML/~~L~~ = 250 ML
250 ML / 12 HR = 20.8 ML/HR

+/- Estimated Ongoing Losses:

1 ML/~~KG~~/HR x 5 ~~KG~~ = 5 ML/HR

CALCULATION OF MAINTENANCE RATE, DEHYDRATION DEFICIT AND ESTIMATED ONGOING LOSSES:

16.6 ML/HR (MAINTENANCE) + 20.8 ML/HR (DEHYDRATION DEFICIT) + 5 ML/HR (ESTIMATED ONGOING LOSSES) = 42.46 ML/HR

CALCULATION WITHOUT ESTIMATED ONGOING LOSSES:

16.6 ML/HR (MAINTENANCE) + 20.8 ML/HR (DEHYDRATION DEFICIT) = 37.4 ML/HR

Remember, if calculating fluids over 12 hours, do not calculate the 80% correction of the dehydration deficit.

TO CALCULATE MAINTENANCE IV FLUID RATES IN ML/KG/DAY

CANINE

0.5xM = 60 ML/KG/DAY X 0.5 = 30 ML/KG/DAY
1xM = 60 ML/KG/DAY
1.5xM = 60 ML/KG/DAY X 1.5 = 90 ML/KG/DAY
2xM = 60 ML/KG/DAY X 2 = 120 ML/KG/DAY
2.5xM = 60 ML/KG/DAY X 2.5 = 150 ML/KG/DAY
3xM = 60 ML/KG/DAY X 3 = 180 ML/KG/DAY

FELINE

0.5xM = 40 ML/KG/DAY X 0.5 = 20 ML/KG/DAY
1xM = 40 ML/KG/DAY
1.5xM = 40 ML/KG/DAY X 1.5 = 60 ML/KG/DAY
2xM = 40 ML/KG/DAY X 2 = 80 ML/KG/DAY
2.5xM = 40 ML/KG/DAY X 2.5 = 100 ML/KG/DAY
3xM = 40 ML/KG/DAY X 3 = 120 ML/KG/DAY

MAINTENANCE FLUID RATE EQUATION USED IN PRACTICE

This fluid rate equation is similar to the rate in the literature stated above but is good for calculating maintenance fluid rates on dogs, cats, kittens and puppies that is more comparable to their actual weights, but does not account for dehydration deficit or ongoing losses. The previously stated process for accounting for these is well documented and superior, but this method is used in practice.

DOG: $((KG)^{0.75})$ x 5.5 ML/KG/HR

CAT: $((KG)^{0.75})$ x 3.3 ML/KG/HR

WEIGHT: 3.3 KG CAT

$((3.3 \text{ KG})^{0.75})$ x 3.3 ML/KG/HR

HOW TO UTILIZE YOUR PHONE CALCULATOR FOR THIS EQUATION

TYPE IN 3.3
THEN HIT x^y
TYPE IN 0.75 THEN EQUALS
THEN MULTIPLY BY 3.3 ML/KG/HR
3.3 ML/~~KG~~/HR x 2.448 ~~KG~~ = 8.08 ML/HR = 1xM

SMARTFLOW FLUID MAINTENANCE RATE EQUATION

This is the equation the SmartFlow utilizes to calculate its maintenance fluid rates.

((1.2 ML/DAY x (KG$^{0.75}$) x 70 KG) / 24 HR/DAY

WEIGHT: 3.3 KG

((1.2 ML/DAY x (3.3$^{0.75}$ KG) x 70 KG) / 24 HR/DAY

((1.2 ML/DAY x (2.448 KG) x 70 KG) / 24 HR/DAY

((2.9376 ML/~~KG~~/DAY) x 70 ~~KG~~) / 24 HR/DAY

205.632 ML/~~DAY~~ / 24 HR/~~DAY~~

8.568 ML/HR = 1xM

Here's how it compares to the 60 ML/KG/DAY equation:

WEIGHT: 3.3 KG

3.3 ~~KG~~ x 60 ML/~~KG~~/DAY = 198 ML/DAY

198 ML/~~DAY~~ / 24 HR/~~DAY~~

8.25 ML/HR

AAHA/AAFP MAINTENANCE FLUID RATE EQUATION USED IN PRACTICE

DOG: $132 \times (BW_{KG})^{0.75}$ ML/DAY

CAT: $80 \times (BW_{KG})^{0.75}$ ML/DAY

WEIGHT: 3.3 KG CAT

$80 \times (3.3)^{0.75}$ ML/DAY

$80 \times (2.448)$ ML/DAY

195 ML/DAY / 24 HR/DAY = 8.16 ML/HR

CHAPTER 2:

BOLUS RATES, SHOCK BOLUSES & INTRAVENOUS FLUID RESUSCITATION

IV FLUID BOLUS RATES

Set your pump's rate, VTBI, and the time will automatically populate letting you know you've done a correct setting.

RATE (mL/hr)
VTBI (VOLUME TO BE INFUSED)

600 mL over 1 hour =
60 ~~mins~~ / 60 ~~mins~~ = 1
600 x 1 = $\underline{600 \text{ mL/hr}}$ = RATE
$\qquad$ 600 mL $\qquad$ VTBI

300 mL over 30 mins =
300 x 2 = $\underline{600}$ = RATE
$\qquad$ 300 $\quad$ VTBI

> The calculations are based upon how many INCREMENTS of 10, 15, 20, 30, and 60 minutes are in 1 hour. Ex. 60 min / 60 min = 1; Ex. 60 min / 15 min = 4

100 mL over 20 mins =
100 x 3 = $\underline{300}$
$\qquad$ 100

150 mL over 15 mins =
150 x 4 = $\underline{600}$
$\qquad$ 150

50 mL over 10 mins =
50 x 6 = $\underline{300}$
$\qquad$ 50

SHOCK BOLUSES & INTRAVENOUS FLUID RESUSCITATION

The term "shock" refers to a syndrome that is clinically recognizable as the result hypoperfusion to the tissues. "Tissue hypoperfusion, if untreated, leads to organ dysfunction and ultimately organ failure. Shock is present in the later stages of most fatal illnesses as circulatory failure is part of the final common pathway leading towards death." (VIN, 2015) To understand the difference between hypovolemia, the most common form of shock, and dehydration, a review is necessary of fluid compartments and how water in the body is lost in these processes.

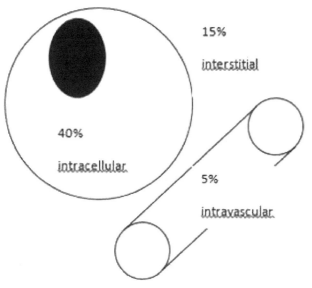

15%

interstitial

40%

intracellular

5%

intravascular

% represents percentage of body weight that is water in different compartments

As can be seen the majority of body water is intracellular and a very small proportion is intravascular.

IMAGE #1 (VIN, 2015)

"Hypovolemia occurs when fluid is lost primarily from the intravascular compartment - a relatively small total loss of fluid has profound physiological consequences with the development of hypovolemic shock. In this circumstance, treatment with fluids centers around rapid replacement of the lost volume to restore tissue perfusion. Conversely dehydration represents fluid loss from all three body fluid compartments. It commonly occurs with more gradual fluid losses where there is time for water to move between body fluid compartments. Total body fluid losses may be much larger than with hypovolemia but as the fluid losses are borne between all the compartments, it has much less profound and immediate physiological effects." (VIN, 2015) Compensated shock is the first stage as blood volume is reduced. Increased heart rate and stroke volume to maintain cardiac output and ultimately tissue perfusion. Decompensated shock is when these mechanisms are successful until a critical point when blood volume is so diminished they are no longer efficacious. Hemodynamic parameters such as blood pressure and bloodwork (i.e. lactate – an anaerobic respiration marker that tells us of tissue perfusion quality), and perfusion parameters are necessary to examine to establish clinical shock. The following perfusion parameter chart should be followed upon each examination of the patient.

PERFUSION PARAMETERS
CANINE

PHYSICAL EXAMINATION FINDINGS	COMPENSATORY SHOCK	EARLY DECOMPENSATORY SHOCK	LATE DECOMPENSATORY SHOCK
Temperature	Normal to low normal (98°F–99°F)[a]	Slight to moderate hypothermia (96°F–98°F)	Moderate to marked hypothermia (<96°F)
Heart rate	Tachycardia (>180 bpm)	Tachycardia (>150 bpm)	Bradycardia (<140 bpm)
Mucous membrane color	Normal to pale (hyperemic in distributive shock)	Pale	Pale to gray/muddy
Capillary refill time	Normal to slightly prolonged (<1 sec; rapid in distributive shock)	Prolonged (<2 sec)	Prolonged (≥2 sec)
Respiratory rate	Tachypnea (>50 breaths/min)	Tachypnea (>50 breaths/min)	Bradypnea
Blood pressure	Slight hypotension to normal (70–80 mm Hg)	Mild to moderate hypotension (50–70 mm Hg)	Marked hypotension refractory to fluid therapy (<60 mm Hg)
Mentation	Responsive	Obtunded	Obtunded to stuporous

Adapted with permission from Thomovsky E, Johnson PA. Shock pathophysiology. *Compend Contin Educ Pract Vet* 2013;35(8):E1-E9.

[a]Values in parentheses are approximate.

FELINE

PHYSICAL EXAMINATION FINDINGS	COMPENSATORY SHOCK	EARLY DECOMPENSATORY SHOCK	LATE DECOMPENSATORY SHOCK
Temperature	Normal to low normal (<97°F)[a]	Slight to moderate hypothermia (<95°F)	Moderate to marked hypothermia (<90°F)
Heart rate	Severe tachycardia (>240 bpm) or mild bradycardia (160–180 bpm)	Moderate tachycardia (>200 bpm) or bradycardia (120–140 bpm)	Mild tachycardia (>180 bpm) or severe bradycardia (<120 bpm)
Mucous membrane color	Pale (hyperemic in distributive shock)	Pale to white	Pale to gray/muddy
Capillary refill time	Normal to slightly prolonged (<1 sec; rapid in distributive shock)	Prolonged (<2 sec)	Prolonged (≥2 sec)
Respiratory rate	Tachypnea (>60 breaths/min)	Tachypnea (>60 breaths/min)	Bradypnea
Blood pressure	Slight hypotension to normal (80–90 mm Hg)	Mild to moderate hypotension (50–80 mm Hg)	Marked hypotension refractory to fluid therapy (<50 mm Hg)
Mentation	Responsive	Obtunded	Obtunded to stuporous

Adapted with permission from Thomovsky E, Johnson PA. Shock pathophysiology. *Compend Contin Educ Pract Vet* 2013;35(8):E1-E9.

[a]Values in parentheses are approximate.

TABLE #2, (TODAY'S VETERINARY NURSE, 2016)

We utilize numerous terms to define an animal's pulse quality. "Bounding" or "hyperkinetic" pulses are tall and narrow and "weak" or "thready" pulses are short and narrow. Bounding pulses are seen in the early stages of hypovolemia whereas weak, thready pulses are seen in late hypovolemic shock. Another parameter we rely on is the electrocardiogram or ECG/EKG. In hypovolemia we witness what is known as sinus tachycardia where the complexes appear normal, but the rate is elevated). "Maximum rate for sinus tachycardia is 220bpm (beats per minute) as at heart rates higher than this cardiac output will actually start to fall as there is insufficient time for ventricular filling." (VIN, 2015)

Before we discuss the treatment of hypovolemia, we need to understand the different types of shock that may present themselves to us. We also need to know and understand contraindications for our patients before treatment begins. We also need to understand the math involved since shock boluses are given in what are called "aliquots" or a portion of a whole volume. Below is how to calculate 1/4 to 1/3 aliquots which are what shock boluses are typically given in since we don't want to fluid overload the patient and we want to see normal parameters with the lowest volume of fluid necessary, however full shock boluses, or boluses equivalent to an animal's blood volume can also be given in very severely compromised cases.

Classification and Consequences of Shock:

HYPOVOLEMIC: Insufficient circulating blood volume and hypoperfusion (ex. Hemorrhaging, Hemoabdomen, et al.)
OBSTRUCTIVE: Extracardiac physical impediment of the great vessels and hypoperfusion (ex. Tamponade/Pericardial Effusion, GDV, Tension Pneumothorax, et al.)
DISTRIBUTIVE: Maldistribution of perfusion and blood volume (ex. SIRS, Sepsis, Anaphylaxis, et al.)
CARDIOGENIC: Primary cardiac pump failure resulting in decreased cardiac output and hypoperfusion. (ex. Myocardial Infarction, Myocarditis, Endocarditis, et al.)

CALCULATING SHOCK BOLUSES

CANINE = 60 - 90 ML/KG TOTAL SHOCK DOSE (LOWER END
UTILIZED IN CARDIAC OR RENAL IMPAIRMENT)
FELINE = 40 - 60 ML/KG TOTAL SHOCK DOSE (LOWER END
UTILIZED IN CARDIAC OR RENAL IMPAIRMENT)

ALWAYS GIVE IN 1/3 TO 1/4 SHOCK DOSE ALIQUOTS

CALCULATE TOTAL SHOCK DOSE AND 1/4 SHOCK DOSE ALIQUOT

OPTION 1 – BY HAND WITH FRACTION
90 ML/KG SHOCK DOSE FOR DOG, THEN 1/4 SHOCK DOSE
ALIQUOT
WEIGHT: 15 KG
TIME: 15 MINUTES

90 ML/KG X 15 KG = 1350 ML TOTAL SHOCK DOSE
90 ML/KG X 1/4 = 90/1 ML/KG X 1/4 = 90/4 = 22.5 ML/KG
22.5 ML/KG X 15 KG = 337.5 ML = 1/4 SHOCK DOSE ALIQUOT =
VTBI
60 MINS / 15 MINS = 4 (4 IS A UNIT OF TIME)
337.5 ML X 4 = 1350 ML/HR = RATE (OVER 15 MINUTES)

RATE: 1350 ML/HR
VTBI: 337.5 ML

OPTION 2 – WITH CALCULATOR WITH DECIMAL
90 ML/KG SHOCK DOSE FOR DOG, THEN 1/4 SHOCK DOSE
ALIQUOT
WEIGHT: 15 KG
TIME: 15 MINUTES

90 ML/~~KG~~ X 15 ~~KG~~ = 1350 ML TOTAL SHOCK DOSE
1350 ML X 0.25 (1/4 IN DECIMAL FORM) = 337.5 ML = 1/4 SHOCK DOSE ALIQUOT = VTBI
60 ~~MINS~~ / 15 ~~MINS~~ = 4 (4 IS A UNIT OF TIME)
337.5 ML X 4 = 1,350 ML/HR = RATE (OVER 15 MINUTES)

RATE: 1,350 ML/HR
VTBI: 337.5 ML

CALCULATE TOTAL SHOCK DOSE AND 1/3 SHOCK DOSE ALIQUOT

OPTION 1 – BY HAND WITH FRACTION
90 ML/KG SHOCK DOSE FOR DOG, THEN 1/3 SHOCK DOSE ALIQUOT
WEIGHT: 15 KG
TIME: 15 MINUTES

90 ML/~~KG~~ X 15 ~~KG~~ = 1350 ML TOTAL SHOCK DOSE
90 ML/KG X 1/3 = 90/1 ML/KG X 1/3 = 90/3 = 30 ML/KG
30 ML/~~KG~~ X 15 ~~KG~~ = 450 ML = 1/3 SHOCK DOSE ALIQUOT = VTBI
60 ~~MINS~~ / 15 ~~MINS~~ = 4 (4 IS A UNIT OF TIME)
450 X 4 = 1,800 ML/HR = RATE (OVER 15 MINUTES)

RATE: 1,800 ML/HR
VTBI: 450 ML

OPTION 2 – WITH CALCULATOR WITH DECIMAL
1/3 IS EQUIVALENT TO 0.333 ON A CALCULATOR

90 ML/KG SHOCK DOSE FOR DOG, THEN 1/3 SHOCK DOSE ALIQUOT
WEIGHT: 15 KG
TIME: 15 MINUTES

90 ML/~~KG~~ X 15 ~~KG~~ = 1350 ML TOTAL SHOCK DOSE
90 ML/KG / 3 = 30 ML/KG
30 ML/~~KG~~ X 15 ~~KG~~ = 450 ML = 1/3 SHOCK DOSE ALIQUOT = VTBI
60 ~~MINS~~ / 15 ~~MINS~~ = 4 (4 IS A UNIT OF TIME)
450 ML X 4 = 1,800 ML/HR = RATE (OVER 15 MINUTES)

RATE: 1,800 ML/HR
VTBI: 450 ML

To bolus on a fluid pump, always set your VTBI to your shock dose aliquot volume and your RATE to 10-30 minutes for crystalloids by multiplying your shock dose aliquot by 6 for 10 minutes, 4 for 15 minutes, 3 for 20 minutes or 2 for 30 minutes, and set that number as your RATE.

Rate

10min x 6
15min x 4
20min x 5
30mix x 2

Other fluid options exist for patients with hypovolemia/hypovolemic shock or profound hypotension such as hypertonic saline or colloids. Hypertonic saline is <u>not</u> given in 1/4 shock bolus aliquots, Hetastarch is given in 1/4 shock bolus aliquots. To calculate the dosage of Hypertonic saline and Hetastarch, follow the instructions below:

HYPERTONIC SALINE FOR CAT
WEIGHT: 5 KG
DOSAGE: 2 ML/KG (2-4 ML/KG CONSERVATIVE DOSING RANGE FOR BOTH DOGS AND CATS)
TIME: OVER 10 MINUTES

2 ML/~~KG~~ X 5 ~~KG~~ = 10 ML HYPERTONIC SALINE = VTBI

TO SET A FLUID PUMP:
60 ~~MINS~~ / 10 ~~MINS~~ = 6 (10 MINUTE INCREMENTS IN 1 HOUR = 6)
10 ML X 6 = 60 ML/HR (6 IS A UNIT OF TIME) = RATE

RATE = 60 ML/HR
VTBI = 10 ML

HYPERTONIC SALINE FOR DOG
WEIGHT: 22.5 KG
DOSAGE: 4 ML/KG (2-4 ML/KG CONSERVATIVE DOSING RANGE FOR BOTH DOGS AND CATS)
TIME: OVER 10 MINUTES

4 ML/~~KG~~ X 22.5 ~~KG~~ = 90 ML HYPERTONIC SALINE = VTBI

TO SET A FLUID PUMP:
60 ~~MINS~~ / 10 ~~MINS~~ = 6 (10 MINUTE INCREMENTS IN 1 HOUR = 6)
90 ML X 6 = 540 ML/HR (6 IS A UNIT OF TIME) = RATE

RATE = 540 ML/HR
VTBI = 90 ML

HETASTARCH FOR CAT

WEIGHT: 4.46 KG

DOSAGE: 10 ML/KG (1/4 SHOCK DOSE ALIQUOT OF 20 ML/KG TOTAL SHOCK DOSE FOR DOGS, 10 ML/KG TOTAL SHOCK DOSE FOR CATS)

TIME: 15 MINUTES

10 ML/~~KG~~ X 4.46 ~~KG~~ = 44.6 ML TOTAL SHOCK DOSE HETASTARCH

TO CALCULATE 1/4 SHOCK BOLUS ALIQUOT:

44.6 ML / 4 = 11.15 ML 1/4 SHOCK BOLUS ALIQUOT = VTBI

TO SET A FLUID PUMP:

60 ~~MINS~~ / 15 ~~MINS~~ = 4 (15 MINUTE INCREMENTS IN 1 HOUR = 4)

11.15 ML X 4 = 44.6 ML/HR (4 IS A UNIT OF TIME) = RATE

RATE: 44.6 ML/HR

VTBI: 11.15 ML

HETASTARCH FOR DOG
WEIGHT: 22.5 KG
DOSAGE: 20 ML/KG (1/4 SHOCK DOSE ALIQUOT OF 20 ML/KG
TOTAL SHOCK DOSE FOR DOGS, 10 ML/KG TOTAL SHOCK DOSE
FOR CATS)
TIME: 15 MINUTES

20 ML/~~KG~~ X 22.5 ~~KG~~ = 450 ML TOTAL SHOCK DOSE HETASTARCH

TO CALCULATE 1/4 SHOCK BOLUS ALIQUOT:
450 ML / 4 = 112.5 ML 1/4 SHOCK BOLUS ALIQUOT = VTBI

TO SET A FLUID PUMP:
60 ~~MINS~~ / 15 ~~MINS~~ = 4 (15 MINUTE INCREMENTS IN 1 HOUR = 4)
112.5 ML X 4 = 450 ML/HR (4 IS A UNIT OF TIME) = RATE

RATE: 450 ML/HR
VTBI: 112.5 ML

OVERVIEW OF RESUSCITATIVE FLUID THERAPY
Alexandre Proulx, DVM, and Deborah Silverstein, DVM, Diplomate ACVECC

Fluid Type	Indications	Dosage Dog	Dosage Cat	Notes
CRYSTALLOID FLUIDS				
Isotonic crystalloids	Patients with fluid-responsive shock; commonly used as initial fluid therapy	90 mL/kg Administer 1/4 to 1/3 of dose; then reassess CV parameters prior to further administration	50 mL/kg	• Examples: 0.9% sodium chloride, lactated Ringer's solution, Normosol-R,* & Plasma-Lyte-A§ • Avoid overzealous use to prevent volume overload and hemodilution of blood constituents
Hypertonic saline	Patients with traumatic brain injury or when rapid intravascular volume expansion is needed	4–7 mL/kg Administer over ≈ 10 min	3–4 mL/kg	• To prolong effect, a hypertonic saline/synthetic colloid mixture can be administered • Contraindicated in patients that are dehydrated, hyperosmolar, or hypokalemic
SYNTHETIC COLLOIDS				
Hydroxyethyl starches	Patients with low colloidal osmotic pressure, increased vascular permeability, or when rapid intravascular volume expansion is needed	20 mL/kg Administer 1/4 to 1/3 of dose; then reassess CV parameters prior to further administration	10 mL/kg	• Of the synthetic colloids available, hydroxyethyl starches are the ones most commonly used in veterinary patients • Use may lead to fluid overload, hemodilution, and coagulation abnormalities
BLOOD PRODUCTS				
Packed red blood cells	Patients with acute anemia & persistent CV instability	10–15 mL/kg Infused over 1–4 H to monitor for adverse reactions (if possible)		**All blood products:** • Blood-typing should be performed before any blood product transfusion. A cross match is recommended if animal has previously received transfusion. • Adverse events include immunologic reactions, electrolyte imbalances, & transmission of disease
Fresh frozen plasma	Patients with prolonged coagulation times	10–15 mL/kg Infused over 1–4 H to monitor for adverse reactions (if possible)		**Fresh frozen plasma:** • Replenishes coagulation factors • Despite being a source of albumin, its colloidal effect is limited due to its relatively low oncotic pressure compared to synthetic colloids
Fresh whole blood	Patients with TCPE, TCPA-induced bleeding, or massive blood loss/surgical candidates with severe TCPE	20–25 mL/kg Infused over 1–4 H to monitor for adverse reactions (if possible)		**Fresh whole blood:** • Same benefits as those of packed red blood cells and fresh frozen plasma combined, but also a source of active platelets

CV = cardiovascular; TCPA = thrombocytopathia; TCPE = thrombocytopenia
* hospira.com
§ baxter.com

This table can be downloaded at **todaysveterinarypractice.com** *and printed for use in your clinic.*

TABLE #3 (Today's Veterinary Practice, 2011)

Resuscitative intravenous fluid therapy is contraindicated for the treatment of cardiogenic shock, but is the cornerstone of therapy for hypovolemic and distributive shock. "Depending on the location of the obstruction, responsiveness to fluid therapy varies with obstructive forms of shock. Resuscitative fluid therapy can be attempted, but treatment of the underlying disorder is ultimately essential (i.e., pericardiocentesis for pericardial effusion causing tamponade)." (Today's Veterinary Practice, 2011) There are four widely recognized types of shock: Hypovolemic, Cardiogenic, Distributive, and Obstructive. There are additional categories of shock that have yet to be universally recognized: Metabolic, Endocrine, Hypoxemic, Neurogenic, Anaphylactic and Septic. However, each of these additional categories can fit into one of the original four universally recognized types.

CHAPTER 3:
DRUG CONCENTRATIONS

DRUG CONCENTRATIONS

The most common formulations of veterinary drugs are utilized for this table. Some drug concentrations may differ from what is listed so be sure to double check the bottle you are working with. – Kind Regards, Management

ACEPROMAZINE	10MG/ML
ALFAXALONE	10MG/ML
AMINOPHYLLINE	25MG/ML
AMPICILLIN	100MG/ML
	250MG/ML
AMPICILLIN SULBACTAM	30MG/ML
	60MG/ML
	375MG/ML
APOMORPHINE	1MG/ML INJ
	3MG/ML INJ
	0.8MG/DROP OPHTH SUSP
ATIPAMEZOLE	5MG/ML
ATROPRINE	1MG/ML
BUPIVICAINE	5MG/ML
BUPRENORPHINE	0.3MG/ML
	0.5MG/ML
	0.6MG/ML
BUTORPHANOL	10MG/ML
CARPROFEN	50MG/ML
CEFAZOLIN	100MG/ML
CEFTAZIDIME	THERE ARE MULTIPLE CONCENTRATIONS FOR THIS MEDICATION AND THE CONCENTRATION IS HIGHLY SITUATIONAL. THE FOLLOWING IS FOR

100MG/ML
CONCENTRATIONS:
1G VIAL:
10ML 0.9% NaCl
10.8 ML WITHDRAWABLE VOLUME RECONSTITUTED
1000 MG / 100 MG/ML = 10 ML
DOSAGE: 30MG/KG Q6H
6.1 KG
30 MG/KG x 6.1 KG = 183 MG
183 MG / 100 MG/ML = 1.83 ML IV SLOW OVER 10 MINUTES THEN FLUSHED WITH 1.83 ML 0.9% NaCl
***CAN ALSO BE CALCULATED TO BE PUT IN BURETROL AND ON SYRINGE PUMP

DEXAMETHASONE	2MG/ML
DEXMEDETOMIDINE	0.5MG/ML
DEX SP	3MG/ML
	4MG/ML
50% DEXTROSE	0.5G/ML
	500MG/ML
DIAZEPAM	5MG/ML
DIPHENHYDRAMINE	50MG/ML
DOXYCYCLINE	100MG/ML
	DILUTE 1:10 TO 10 MG/ML
ENROFLOXACIN	2.27% = 22.7 MG/ML
EPINEPHRINE	1MG/ML
EUTHASOL	390MG/ML
FENTANYL	50MCG/ML

FUROSEMIDE	50MG/ML
HYDROMORPHONE	2MG/ML
KCL	2MEQ/ML
KETAMINE	100MG/ML
LEVETIRACETAM	100MG/ML
2% LIDOCAINE	20MG/ML
20% MANNITOL	20% = 200MG/ML
MAROPITANT	10MG/ML
MELOXICAM	5MG/ML INJ
	1.5MG/ML PO
METHADONE	10MG/ML
METHOCARBAMOL	100MG/ML
METOCLOPRAMIDE	5MG/ML
METRONIDAZOLE	5MG/ML
MIDAZOLAM	5MG/ML
MORPHINE	4MG/ML
N-ACETYLCYSTEINE	50MG/ML
	DILUTE TO 5% CONC.
	(200MG/ML AMPOULE)
	DILUTE 1:4 (5 PARTS)
	WITH 0.45% NaCl,
	STERILE H2O OR 5%
	DEXTROSE AS SPECIFIED
	BY DVM
NOREPINEPHRINE	1MG/ML
ONDANSETRON	2MG/ML
PANTOPRAZOLE	4MG/ML
PHENOBARBITAL	100MG/ML
PRAZIQUANTEL	56.8MG/ML
PREDNISOLONE	20MG/ML
	3MG/ML = 15MG/5ML
PROPOFOL	10MG/ML
TILETAMINE	100MG/ML
VASOPRESSIN	20U/ML
XYLAZINE	20MG/ML

CHAPTER 4: ALGEBRA REVIEW

ALGEBRA REVIEW

Not everyone remembers their high school or college math classes, and it's totally okay! Math was never my strong suit in school but once I started working in the veterinary field and started learning medical math, algebra and statistics became extremely easy for me. and eventually I ended up getting A's in both of my college algebra and statistics courses, and I hope you have the same success. So, with that being said, let's learn some basic algebra!

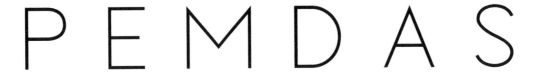

Please Excuse My Dear Aunt Sally

Parentheses

Exponents

Multiplication

Division

Addition

Subtraction

This is one of the most important rules to remember when working with constant rate infusion equations and drug calculations. As you will see, keeping your units of measure in check is also of supreme importance.

QUICK ALGEBRA REVIEW

Just cancel out your units of measure that are the same! Carry over the unit of measure that is remaining. This can become difficult to come to the correct answer if you are using mL/kg/day, have to convert days to hrs, or if you just are working off of someone else's math (double checking for instance), and they don't utilize the appropriate units of measure in their work. **Always** write the appropriate units of measure and cancel out as you go. This book displays its math in linear algebraic format rather than dimensional analysis. This format is easier to comprehend for beginners as well as seasoned medical mathematicians.

EXAMPLES

10 mg / 20 mg/mL

10 ~~mg~~ / 20 ~~mg~~/mL

= 0.5 mL

50 mL/~~kg~~/day x 41.31 ~~kg~~ = 2065.5 mL/day

2065.5 mL/~~day~~ / 24 hr/~~day~~

= 86 mL/hr

20 ~~mEq~~/L / 2 ~~mEq~~/mL

= 10 mL/L

CHAPTER 5: TOXICOLOGY

TOXICOLOGY

A primary reason for emergency room visits for pets is ingestion or contact with a toxic substance. It is the doctor's job to identify the substance, diagnose the condition, order diagnostics, interpret the results, and then prescribe treatment. It is the technician's job to get a patient history and vitals upon presentation, round the doctor, perform diagnostics and labwork, administer the patient's treatments, and then continually monitor the patient's status and vitals, informing the doctor of any changes. These cases can change rapidly, so paying close attention to these patients is vital.

The following table will guide you via antidote, not toxicity, as there are far too many toxicities to name. However, common antidote and toxicity/indication information is included in this table along with contraindications, antidote drug dosages for both dogs and cats, and administration and storage information.

COMMON VETERINARY TOXICITIES, ANTIDOTES, DOSAGES AND ADMINISTRATION, STORAGE AND CONTRAINDICATIONS

TABLE #4 (Hare, Post, and Oehme, n.d.)

ANTIDOTE	TOXICITY/INDICATION	DOSAGE	ADMINISTRATION AND STORAGE	CONTRAINDICATIONS
INTRALIPIDS (INTRAVENOUS FAT EMULSION) IFE'S OR (INTRAVENOUS LIPID EMULSION) ILE'S CONC. 20%	ANTIDOTE FOR LIPOPHILIC DRUG MOLECULES: AMLODIPINE, VERAPAMIL, BETAXOLOL, BUPROPION, BACLOFEN, CARVEDIOL, CYCLIC ANTIDEPRESSANTS, METOPROLOL, ORGANOPHOSPHATES, PROPRANOLOL, BROMADIOLONE, DIPHENHYDRAMINE, QUETIAPINE, DILITIAZEM, DFIHYDROPYRIDINES, COCAINE, IAMOTRIDINE, IVERMECTIN, PEST/INSECTICIDES, MALATHION, OLANZIPINE, ANTIPSYCHOTICS, SSRI'S, CARBAMATE, METHAMPHETAMINE, DEXTROAMPHETAMINE, BROMETHALIN, LIDOCAINE, PERMETHRIN, IBUPROFEN, CHOLECALCIFEROL, MACROLYTIC LACTONES	DOGS: BOLUS: 1.5ML/KG-4ML/KG IV OVER 1 MIN FOLLOWED BY CRI: 0.25-0.5ML/KG/MIN IV OVER 30-60 MINS *CAN REPEAT BOLUS IF NO SIGNS OF IMPROVEMENT IN 1-4 HOURS. INTERMITTENT BOLUS DOSING: 1.5ML/KG IV Q4-6H FOR 24H OR *FOR CONTINUOUS CLINICAL SIGNS: CRI: 0.5ML/KG/HR IV UNTIL IMPROVEMENT *IF CLINICAL SIGNS DO NOT IMPROVE, DISCONTINUE ILE'S CATS: BOLUS: 1.5MLS/KG-4ML/KG IV OVER 1 MIN FOLLOWED BY CRI: 0.25ML/KG/MIN IV OVER 30-60 MINS *CAN REPEAT BOLUS IF NO SIGNS OF IMPROVEMENT IN 1-4 HOURS. INTERMITTENT BOLUS DOSING: 1.5ML/KG IV Q4-6H FOR 24H OR *FOR CONTINUOUS CLINICAL SIGNS: CRI: 0.5ML/KG/HR IV UNTIL IMPROVEMENT *IF CLINICAL SIGNS DO NOT IMPROVE, DISCONTINUE ILE'S	DEDICATED PERIPHERAL IV CATHETER WITHOUT BIFURCATOR OR TRIFURCATOR IN PLACE. CENTRAL LINE NOT NECESSARY. CANNOT RUN IN SAME LINE AS IVF. ON FLUID PUMP OR SYRINGE PUMP GOOD FOR 24 HOURS AFTER OPENING SHOULD NOT BE STORED ABOVE 77°F/25°C DO NOT FREEZE	DISTURBANCES OF NORMAL FAT METABOLISM SUCH AS PATHOLOGIC HYPERLIPIDEMIA, LIPOID NEPHROSIS, OR ACUTE PANCREATITIS IF ACCOMPANIED BY HYPERLIPIDEMIA (BAXTER, 2015)

ANTIDOTE	TOXICITY/INDICATION	DOSAGE	ADMINISTRATION AND STORAGE	CONTRAINDICATIONS
N-ACETYLCYSTEINE CONC. 20% 50MG/ML DILUTE TO 5% CONC. 200MG/ML AMPOULE) MUCOLYTIC WHICH REDUCES DISULFIDE LINKAGE RESTORING GLUTATHIONE LEVELS BY ACTING AS A *S* SUBSTITUTE IN ACETAMINOPHEN POISONING.	ANTIDOTE FOR ACETAMINOPHEN/NSAID TOXICOSIS ASCORBIC ACID, METHYLENE BLUE, BICARBONATE, ACTIVATED CHARCOAL, OMEPRAZOLE, PANTOPRAZOLE, MISOPROSTOL.	DOGS: 140 - 180 MG/KG IV FOLLOWED BY 70-75 MG/KG IV or PO q6h CATS: 140 MG/KG IV FOLLOWED BY 70-75 MG/KG IV or PO q6h	200MG/ML DILUTE TO 5% CONC. (50MG/ML) DILUTE 1:4 (5 PARTS) WITH 0.45% NaCl, STERILE H2O OR 5% DEXTROSE AS SPECIFIED BY DVM.. **TO CALCULATE PLEASE SEE N-ACETYLCYSTEINE PAGE 95**	
FLUMAZENIL 0.1 MG/ML CONC.	REVERSAL FOR BENZODIAZEPINE OVERDOSE AND TOXICOSIS DIAZEPAM, LORAZEPAM, ALPRAZOLAM, ETHYL ALCOHOL POISONING	DOGS AND CATS: 0.01-0.2MG/KG SLOWLY IV PRN OR 0.05MG/KG/HR IV DRIP. DOGS, CATS: DOSE NOT TO EXCEED 2MG.	BOLUS SLOWLY IV PRN OR GIVE AS A CRI AT 0.05MG/KG/HR	MONITOR FOR EFFICACY AND SEIZURE INDUCTION.

ANTIDOTE	TOXICITY/INDICATION	DOSAGE	ADMINISTRATION AND STORAGE	CONTRAINDICATIONS
NALOXONE *0.4 MG/ML STANDARD CONC. 1 MG/ML CONC. 10 ML VIAL OPIOID ANTAGONIST/PURE ANALOG COMPETES WITH AND DISPLACES NARCOTIC AT RECEPTOR SITES (MU, KAPPA, AND SIGMA) USED IN NARCOTIC AND NARCOTIC-LIKE POISONINGS	REVERSAL FOR OPIOIDS POOR REVERSAL AGENT FOR BUPRENORPHINE BUTORPHANOL, ALFENTANIL, BELLADONNA (ATROPUS), BUPRENORPHINE, PENTAZOCINE, CAPTOPRIL, NALABUPHINE, CLONIDINE, CODEINE, HEROIN, DXM, ATROPINE, DIPHENOXYLATE, FENTANYL CITRATE, GHBA, GUANFACINE, HYDROCODONE, HOMATROPINE, KETOBEMIDONE, LEVOMETHADYL, LEVOPHANOL TARTRATE, LISINOPRIL, LOPERAMIDE, MEPERIDINE, METHADONE, MORPHINE, NITROUS OXIDE, OPIUM ALKALOIDS, OPIUM TINCTURE, OXYCODONE, OXYMORPHONE, PAREGORIC, PROPOXYPHENE, SULFENTANIL, VALPROIC ACID, ZIPEPROL, JIMSONWEED (DATURA), JESSAMINE (CESTRUM), HENBANE (HYOSCYAMUS), POPPY (PAPAVER)	DOGS AND CATS: 0.01-0.05MG/KG IV SLOWLY PRN DRUG EFFECT IS OF SHORT DURATION (30-60 MINUTES) YOU MUST THEREFORE CONTINUOUSLY MONITOR FOR RECURRENT ADVERSE EFFECTS	BOLUS SLOWLY IV PRN	OPIOID DEPENDENCE HYPERSENSITIVITIES CARDIAC ABNORMALITIES
DIPHENHYDRAMINE 50MG/ML CONC. 1 ML VIAL ANTIHISTAMINE SEDATIVE ANTICHOLINERGIC ANTIEMETIC REVERSE TOXOID AND TOXIN INDUCED EXTRAPYRAMIDAL EFFECTS	ANTIDOTE FOR HISTAMINE REACTION, POISONINGS AND DRUG OVERDOSE PACLITAXEL, MONOSODIUM, GLUTAMATE, ANTIVENIN, HALOPERIDOL, PHENOTHIAZINE, DERIVATIVES AND TRANQUILIZERS (ACEPROMAZINE).	DOGS: 0.5-4.0 MG/KG IV, IM PRN CATS: 0.5-1.0 MG/KG IV, IM PRN	IV, IM PRN IF GIVING IV: DILUTE 1:1 WITH SALINE FOR IV INFUSION OVER 10-15 MINUTES BUT **CONFIRM WITH DVM FIRST** IM ROUTE PREFERRED	

UAA GEL CALCULATION

DOSAGE GIVEN BY DOCTOR: 25 G
CONCENTRATION: 120 MG/ML

25 G X 1000 MG/G = 25,000 MG
25,000 MG / 120 MG/ML = 208.3 ML UAA GEL

TOXIBAN WITH AND WITHOUT SORBITOL

DOSAGE RANGE: 5 TO 10 ML PER POUND
WEIGHT: 18.9 KG = 41.6 LB
DOSAGE UTILIZED: 5 ML/LB

41.5 LB X 5 ML/LB = 208 ML

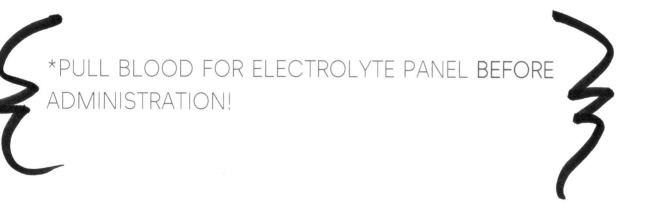

*PULL BLOOD FOR ELECTROLYTE PANEL **BEFORE** ADMINISTRATION!

TOXIBAN SUSPENSION WITH AND WITHOUT SORBITOL

PET POISON HELPLINE AND ASPCA POISON CONTROL TYPICALLY RECOMMEND DOSES OF 1-3 G/KG OF ACTIVATED CHARCOAL, HERE IS HOW TO CALCULATE TOXIBAN SUSPENSION IN G/KG

ORDER: 1 G/KG
WEIGHT: 20 KG
CONC.: 10.4% ACTIVATED CHARCOAL
BOTTLE VOLUME: 240 ML

10.4% SOLUTION = 10.4 G / 100 ML – "10.4 G PER 100 ML" = 10,400 MG / 100 ML = 104 MG/ML = CONC.

1 G/KG = 1000 MG/KG

1000 MG/~~KG~~ X 20 ~~KG~~ = 20,000 MG
20,000 ~~MG~~ / 104 ~~MG~~/ML = 192 ML

TO FIND ML/KG:

192 ML / 20 KG = 9.6 ML/KG

ON LABEL DOSING OF TOXIBAN SUSPENSION WITH AND WITHOUT SORBITOL

TOXIBAN LABELS SUGGEST DOSES OF 5-10 ML/LB OR 10-20 ML/KG. THESE DOSES ARE NOT EQUIVALENT. **CONFIRM WITH DVM** WHICH DOSING THEY WOULD LIKE TO UTILIZE.

EXAMPLE:

DOSAGE: 10-20 ML/KG OR 5-10 ML/LB
WEIGHT: 20 KG = 44 LB

10 ML/~~KG~~ X 20 ~~KG~~ = 200 ML

11 ML/~~KG~~ X 20 ~~KG~~ = 220 ML = 5 ML/LB X 44 LB = 220 ML

20 ML/~~KG~~ X 20 ~~KG~~ = 400 ML

22 ML/~~KG~~ X 20 ~~KG~~ = 440 ML = 10 ML/LB X 44 LB = 440 ML

*SO WE CAN SEE THAT DOSING CALCULATIONS AND RECOMMENDATIONS ARE VARIABLE FOR TOXIBAN. THE 1 G/KG RECOMMENDATION FROM POISON CONTROL IS EQUAL TO 192 ML AND 9.6 ML/KG WHILE ON LABEL DOSING IS HIGHER. THIS DRUG CAN INCREASE SODIUM CONCENTRATIONS SO AN ELECTROLYTE PANEL MUST BE RUN PRIOR TO ADMINISTRATION AND A JUDICIOUS BUT CLINICALLY EFFECTIVE DOSAGE SHOULD BE UTILIZED. CONFIRM ALL DOSAGES AND FINAL TOTAL VOLUME WITH DVM BEFORE ADMINISTERING.

CHAPTER 6:
RECOVER PROTOCOL INTRATRACHEAL DRUG ADMINISTRATION & ADVANCED VENOUS ACCESS

RECOVER PROTOCOL INTRATRACHEAL DRUG ADMINISTRATION

RECOVER clinical guidelines

Appendix II

CPR drug doses. BLS, basic life support; CPA, cardiopulmonary arrest; CRI, constant rate infusion; IV, intravenous; IO, intraosseus; IT, intratracheal; PCA, postcardiac arrest; PEA, pulseless electrical activity; VF, ventricular fibrillation; VT, ventricular tachycardia.

	Drug	Common concentration	Dose/route	Comments
Arrest	Epinephrine (low dose)	1 mg/mL (1:1000)	0.01 mg/kg IV/IO 0.02–0.1 mg/kg IT	Administer every other BLS cycle for asystole/PEA. Consider increasing dose 2–10× and diluting with saline or sterile water for IT administration
	Epinephrine (high dose)	1 mg/mL (1:1000)	0.1 mg/kg IV/IO/IT	Start with low dose. Consider high dose for prolonged (>10 min) CPR
	Vasopressin	20 U/mL	0.8 U/kg IV/IO 1.2 U/kg IT	Administer every other BLS cycle. Increase dose for IT use.
	Atropine	0.54 mg/mL	0.04 mg/kg IV/IO 0.15–0.2 mg/kg IT	May repeat every other BLS cycle during CPR. Recommended in animals with bradycardic arrests and/or known or suspected high vagal tone. Increase dose for IT use.
	Bicarbonate	1 mEq/mL	1 mEq/kg IV/IO	For prolonged (>10–15 min) CPR or in PCA phase to treat severe metabolic acidosis. Contraindicated if patient is hypoventilating.
Antiarrhythmic	Amiodarone	50 mg/mL	5 mg/kg IV/IO	Use for refractory VF/pulseless VT. Has been associated with allergic reactions/hypotension in dogs.
	Lidocaine	20 mg/mL	2 mg/kg slow IV/IO push (1–2 min)	Use for refractory VF/pulseless VT *only* if amiodarone is not available.
Reversals	Naloxone	0.4 mg/mL	0.04 mg/kg IV/IO	To reverse opioids
	Flumazenil	0.1 mg/mL	0.01 mg/kg IV/IO	To reverse benzodiazepines
	Atipamezole	5 mg/mL	100 µg/kg IV/IO	To reverse α2 agonists. Note that this dose is based on a 10 µg/kg dexmedetomidine dose. If a higher dose of dexmedetomidine was administered, increase this dose accordingly.

(TABLE #5. RECOVER Clinical Guidelines, 2012)

The use of the intratracheal route may be considered for administration of drugs in cats and dogs in which intravenous or intraosseous access is not feasible. Epinephrine (Adrenaline), Vasopressin, Naloxone, Lidocaine, or Atropine may be given via this route (NAVEL is the acronym you should commit to memory to remember these drugs). If the intratracheal route is utilized for drug administration during cardiopulmonary resuscitation efforts, the dose should be increased 2-10x the intravenous dosage, then drugs should be diluted in 5 to 10mL of saline or sterile water and administered via a catheter longer than the endotracheal tube, such as a patient appropriate sized red rubber, and 5-6 quick breaths with an Ambu bag/bag valve mask should be given to help the drugs enter the patient's circulation. Diluting the drugs creates one single action down the ET tube and is preferred. You can also pre-draw up 6 and 12 mL syringes of saline to follow drug dosages down the ET tube with a red rubber catheter. Attempts at venous access should continue with the consideration of intraosseous catheterization or a venous cutdown procedure if continually unable to get traditional venous access.

Advanced Vascular Access: Intraosseous Catheters Including

EZ-IO *Article by Anne Lindsay, LVT, CVPP, CCRP, CCMT, FFCP, OACM, VTS (Clinical Practice – Canine/Feline)*

Indications: Small or flat veins that are due to: patient size (neonate/pediatric) or small mammals/exotics, vasoconstriction, patient with cardiovascular collapse, hypotensive patient, patients in shock, arrested patient in need of CPR, patients with peripheral edema, patients in status epilepticus, patients who are morbidly obese, patients with generalized wounds, burns or bite wounds surrounding common peripheral veins

Effectiveness: Fluid administration and rehydration are equal to that of peripheral and central catheters. However, administration of drugs take slightly longer to reach peak effect; however, they last longer in duration due to the marrow consistency and contents. Can sample blood from the IO catheter; however, blood values can be affected – mainly: potassium, glucose, and pH (acid/base status). iSTAT machines are most amenable to small volume blood draws from IO catheters.

Advantage: Because it is placed into the bone marrow, the bone does not collapse. Therefore, once trained you may be more successful in placing an IO catheter during CPR then a peripheral IV catheter.

Disadvantage: Can only be left in recumbent patients for only up to 72 hours (most patients will have it in 2-12 hours. Once patients are up and moving then ideally switch to an intravenous catheter.

Complications: Osteomyelitis (most common), introduction of bacteria into the bone marrow, bone fracture, extravasation, compartment syndrome (muscle, nerve, vessel damage) - rare

Site and Needle Type/Gauge Determination: Patient size, body conformation, level of ambulation/mobility, user preference

Types of Intraosseous Catheter: Hypodermic needle (24g -to 16ga), bone marrow needle, IO infusion needle, automated device (electric or spring loaded). Example: EZ-IO drill. *For EZ-IO catheters the needle gauge is always the same (15g). However, the length of the needle varies between 3 sizes (15mm, 25mm, 45mm).*

Site Placement:

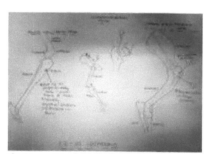

© Anne Lindsay, 2022

Full size image on last page

EZ-IO catheter:

Medial Proximal Tibia *(more common in larger dogs without previous surgeries here i.e. TPLO or TTA)*

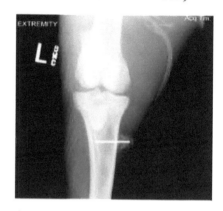

Greater Tubercle of the Humerus *(more common in cats and small dogs)*

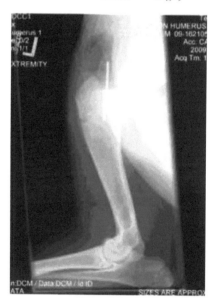

Advanced Vascular Access: Intraosseous Catheters Including

EZ-IO *Article by Anne Lindsay, LVT, CVPP, CCRP, CCMT, FFCP, OACM, VTS (Clinical Practice – Canine/Feline)*

Intertrochanteric Fossa of the Femur

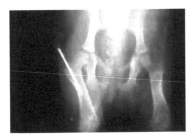

Wings of the Ilium or Ischium

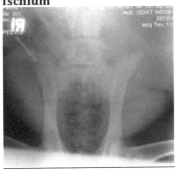

Hypodermic needles:

Intertrochanteric Fossa *(common for neonates/pediatrics)*

Greater Tubercle of the Humerus *(common in exotics)*

Bone marrow needle:

Greater Tubercle of the Humerus *(large dogs)*

Contraindications:
Depending on site placement

Medial Proximal Tibia

Previous TTA surgery
Previous TPLO surgery
Previous extracapsular repair
Fracture or history of fracture of the tibia
Skin that has lacerations, abrasions, burns, dermatitis, ectoparasites, fungal or bacterial infection
Bone Neoplasia
Osteomyelitis

Greater Tubercle of the Humerus

Fracture or history of fracture of the humerus
Skin that has lacerations, abrasions, burns, dermatitis, ectoparasites, fungal or bacterial infection
Bone Neoplasia
Osteomyelitis

Intertrochanteric Fossa of the Femur

Previous THR
Previous FHO surgery
Fracture or history of fracture of the femur or acetabulum
Skin that has lacerations, abrasions, burns, dermatitis, ectoparasites, fungal or bacterial infection
Bone Neoplasia
Osteomyelitis

Wings of the Ilium or Ischium

Fracture or history of fracture of the pelvis
Bone Neoplasia
Osteomyelitis

Site Preparation: Shave the skin of the insertion site, scrub if not in an emergent situation (if this is a **CPR case** - just shave and spray 2% chlorohexidine/70% isopropyl alcohol on), stab incision *(user preference)*

Procedure:

For EZ-IO: *(I recommend only placing them in the medial proximal tibia or greater tubercle of the humerus due to the difficultly of placement in the trochanteric fossa, ilium and ischium.)*

Shave the fur from the insertion site of choice and quickly disinfect the skin. Can make a stab incision (user preference). **If the fur is not shaved then it will twist around the needle as you are drilling!**

Choose the appropriate size needle set depending on the age, and size of your patient and the insertion site of choice. Attach the needle set to the driver; there is a magnet that holds the needle in place.

Grasp the power driver with your dominant hand. Locate the site of insertion and firmly push the needle through the skin until bone is reached. Holding the skin taut with the other hand, depress the trigger on the gun to drive the needle through the bone into the medullary cavity. **(It will sound like a power drill!)** Once the base of the needle is against the skin, release the trigger of the gun. Detach the gun from the needle base.

Advanced Vascular Access: Intraosseous Catheters Including

EZ-IO *Article by Anne Lindsay, LVT, CVPP, CCRP, CCMT, FFCP, OACM, VTS (Clinical Practice – Canine/Feline)*

Remove the stylet by twisting the upper plastic portion off, revealing the lumen of the catheter.

Attach a saline filled t-set. Aspirate back. *If no marrow rich blood is aspirated it does not necessarily mean it is a failed placement.* If no blood or bone marrow contents appear within the line, flush a small volume of saline to clear any potential bony plugs from the catheter. Then try re-aspirating. *Palpate the opposite side of the bone during the saline flush to determine if there is any extravasation; if there is it may mean that you through the cortex on the other side of the bone. Also, keep in mind that there will be more resistance to administering drugs and fluids IO compared to IV.*

For hypodermic or bone marrow needles:

Direct the needle medially into the intertrochanteric fossa in between the greater and lesser trochanter, or angle distally into the greater tubercle, rotating clockwise and counterclockwise while placing firm pressure until a release of resistance is felt.

*To secure hypodermic or bone marrow needles place a "butterfly" tape around the hub of the catheter. Then suture the tape to the skin.

Confirmation: Firmness of insertion site, catheter/needle moves with the limb (for hypodermic or bone marrow needles), aspiration of bone marrow contents, saline infusion has low resistance, little back-pressure, and you do not observe a subcutaneous "bleb"

Pain control: Administration of opioids, NSAIDs, Gabapentin, and injectable anesthetic such as Lidocaine

Maintenance: Routine observation every 2 hours

Avoid: Hypertonic fluids, high volume fluids under high pressure

References:

Kenichiro Yagi. Advanced Vascular Access – Intraosseous Catheters. VETgirl – Real Life Rounds, 2017.

Intraosseous Catheterization. EZ-IO. Vet Bloom, 2016
Soren Boysen. Intraosseous Fluid Devices. VIN, 2014

Advanced Vascular Access: Intraosseous Catheters Including

EZ-IO *Article by Anne Lindsay, LVT, CVPP, CCRP, CCMT, FFCP, OACM, VTS (Clinical Practice – Canine/Feline)*

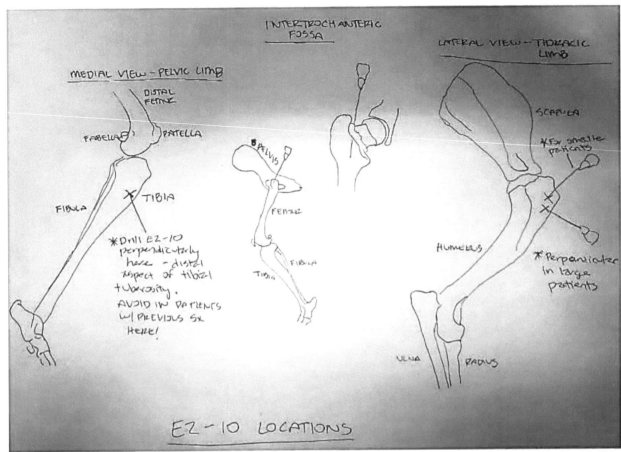

© Anne Lindsay, 2022

CHAPTER 7:
CONSTANT RATE
INFUSIONS

CONSTANT RATE INFUSIONS / CRI'S

A CRI is utilized when a patient requires a drug that is steadily dosed in a given rate over time. It is too labor intensive to have a Veterinary Technician slowly push all drugs, and sometimes a drug needs to be administered in an equivalent portion through a patient's therapy. This is usually achieved by using a syringe pump or a fluid pump. There are many different CRI calculations for the different drugs that can be utilized for infusion therapy. The following is a collection of CRI's with the math included since we do not routinely utilize computer calculators in the veterinary field, as they do in human medicine. We still work the math in most cases. It's good experience to know this kind of math, as it will help you with other drug calculations as well. The first thing you need to do when approaching a CRI is to write down your Order, Weight, Rate, Fluids, and Concentration. This will allow you to have all of the necessary information to complete the algebraic formulas that follow.

One of the simplest CRI's is for Midazolam. It is good practice to write whether a drug is light sensitive, precipitates, or binds to plastic on your CRI to help you remember to take steps to protect the medication or to bleed your line (50 cc's is usually recommended).

Light sensitive indicates that ultraviolet light can cause photodegradation to sensitive medications in a solution through oxidation, hydrolysis, and loss of potency.

Precipitation means that crystallization can occur and binds to plastic means that a medication can adhere to plastic or PVC so we bleed the line to ensure the plastic is thoroughly coated prior to running the medication.

Here is how a **CRI** is set up:

LIGHT SENSITIVE – Indicate if your drug is light sensitive on the label
PRECIPITATES – Indicate if your drug will precipitate in the line on the label

BINDS TO PLASTIC – Indicate if your drug will bind to plastic on the label and if it must be bled 50mL first

Indicate on your label whether your CRI is STRAIGHT or DILUTE.

A **straight** CRI is just the drug (straight) with no other fluid to dilute it in.

A **diluted** CRI is the drug (diluted) in a volume of fluid and gives you a new concentration.

Order: Your Doctor's Order
Weight: Patient's weight in KG
Rate: How you will deliver your drug over time. Either ML/HR, ML/KG/HR or ML/KG/DAY. If unknown place a variable here.
Fluids: This is if your drug is diluted or added to a fluid bag, it is the amount of fluid your drug is diluted in. Either ML or L. If unknown place a variable here.
Time: Timeframe drug needs to last. Either in MIN or HR. If unknown place a variable here.
Concentration: Your Drug's Concentration

DIAZEPAM CRI (STRAIGHT – MG/KG/HR)
LIGHT SENSITIVE / PRECIPITATES / BINDS TO PLASTIC

ORDER: 2 MG/KG/HR
WEIGHT: 3.6 KG
RATE: X
TIME: 10 HR
CONC.: 5 MG/ML

CALCULATE YOUR CRI:

2 MG/~~KG~~/HR X 3.6 ~~KG~~ = 7.2 MG/HR

ORDER X WEIGHT = MG/HR
WE WANT TO START WITH THE ORDER AND MULTIPLY BY THE
WEIGHT TO CANCEL OUT KG AND GET TO MG/HR

7.2 MG/~~HR~~ X 10 ~~HR~~ = 72 MG

MG/HR X TIME = MG
THEN WE WANT TO FACTOR IN TIME AND CANCEL OUT OUR HR TO
GET MG BY ITSELF

72 ~~MG~~ / 5 ~~MG~~/ML = 14.4 ML DIAZEPAM

MG / CONC = ML (TOTAL VOLUME)
THEN WE WANT TO DIVIDE OUR MG BY OUR CONC TO GET TO
OUR TOTAL VOLUME IN ML

CALCULATE YOUR RATE:

14.4 ML / 10 HR = 1.44 ML/HR = RATE = X

ML (TOTAL VOLUME) / TIME = RATE = X

WE NEED TO FIGURE OUT OUR RATE NOW THAT WE HAVE OUR TOTAL VOLUME AND DIVIDE BY OUR TIME TO GET ML/HR

ORDER: 2 MG/KG/HR
WEIGHT: 3.6 KG
RATE: 1.44 ML/HR
TIME: 10 HR
CONC.: 5 MG/ML

TO SET YOUR SYRINGE PUMP, CHOOSE THE **ML/HR OPTION** AND ENTER **1.44 ML/HR** RATE AND **20 ML** SYRINGE SIZE AND YOUR PUMP IS NOW SET FOR A 10 HOUR INFUSION OF DIAZEPAM.

Diazepam cannot be diluted as precipitation will occur in 0.9% NaCl.

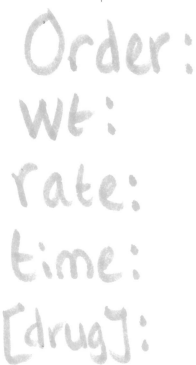

Order:
Wt:
rate:
time:
[drug]:

MIDAZOLAM CRI (STRAIGHT — MG/KG/HR)
LIGHT SENSITIVE

ORDER: 0.2 MG/KG/HR
WEIGHT: 30.3 KG
RATE: X
TIME: 10 HR
CONC.: 5 MG/ML

0.2 MG/~~KG~~/HR X 30.3 ~~KG~~ = 6.06 MG/HR

ORDER X WEIGHT = MG/HR
WE WANT TO START WITH THE ORDER AND MULTIPLY BY THE
WEIGHT TO CANCEL OUT KG AND GET TO MG/HR

6.06 MG/~~HR~~ X 10 ~~HR~~ = 60.6 MG MIDAZOLAM

MG/HR X TIME = MG
THEN WE WANT TO FACTOR IN TIME AND CANCEL OUT OUR HR TO
GET MG BY ITSELF

60.6 ~~MG~~ / 5 ~~MG~~/ML = 12.12 ML MIDAZOLAM (TOTAL VOLUME)

MG / CONC = ML (TOTAL VOLUME)
THEN WE WANT TO DIVIDE OUR MG BY OUR CONC TO GET TO
OUR TOTAL VOLUME IN ML

12.12 ML MIDAZOLAM / 10 HR = 1.212 ML/HR = RATE = X

ML (TOTAL VOLUME) / TIME = RATE = X

WE NEED TO FIGURE OUT OUR RATE NOW THAT WE HAVE OUR TOTAL VOLUME AND DIVIDE BY OUR TIME TO GET ML/HR

ORDER: 0.2 MG/KG/HR
WEIGHT: 30.3 KG
RATE: 1.212 ML/HR
TIME: 10 HR
CONC.: 5 MG/ML

TO SET YOUR SYRINGE PUMP, CHOOSE THE **ML/HR OPTION** AND ENTER **1.2 ML/HR** RATE AND **12 ML** SYRINGE SIZE AND YOUR PUMP IS NOW SET FOR A 10 HOUR INFUSION OF MIDAZOLAM.

Now let's up the ante and try the diluted Midazolam version without as much help!

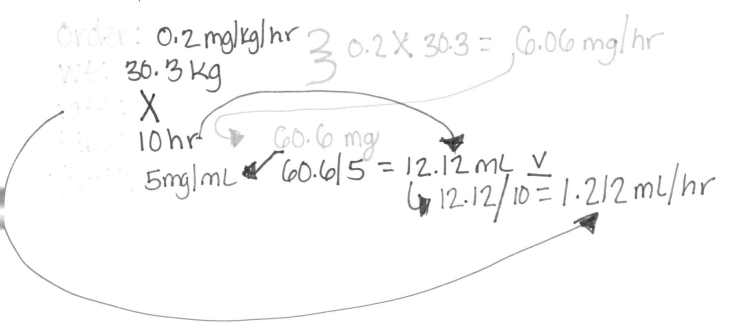

Order: 0.2 mg/kg/hr
We: 30.3 kg
X
10 hr
5 mg/mL

3 0.2 × 30.3 = 6.06 mg/hr

60.6 mg

60.6/5 = 12.12 mL
12.12/10 = 1.212 mL/hr

MIDAZOLAM CRI (DILUTE — MG/KG/HR)

LIGHT SENSITIVE

ORDER: 0.2 MG/KG/HR
WEIGHT: 30.3 KG
RATE: RUN AT 2 ML/HR
FLUID: X
TIME: 10 HR
CONC.: 5 MG/ML

CALCULATE YOUR CRI:

0.2 MG/~~KG~~/HR X 30.3 ~~KG~~ = 6.06 MG/HR
ORDER X WEIGHT = MG/HR

6.06 MG/~~HR~~ X 10 ~~HRS~~ = 60.6 MG
MG/HR X TIME = MG

60.6 ~~MG~~ / 5 ~~MG~~/ML = 12.12 MLS MIDAZOLAM
MG / CONC = ML (VOLUME OF DRUG)

DILUTION:

2 ML/~~HR~~ X 10 ~~HR~~ = 20 ML TOTAL VOLUME
RATE X TIME = X = ML (TOTAL VOLUME)

20 ML – 12.12 ML = 7.88 ML 0.9% NaCl = X = FLUIDS
TOTAL VOLUME – VOLUME OF DRUG = X = FLUIDS

Great job! The next CRI that is easiest to understand is Lasix/Furosemide - Dilute.

LASIX/FUROSEMIDE CRI (DILUTE — MG/KG/HR)
LIGHT SENSITIVE

ORDER: 1 MG/KG/HR
WEIGHT: 10.5 KG
RATE: RUN AT 1 ML/HR
FLUID: X AMOUNT OF 0.9% NaCl
TIME: 6 HR
CONC.: 50 MG/ML

CALCULATE YOUR CRI:

1 MG/~~KG~~/HR x 10.5 ~~KG~~ = 10.5 MG/HR
10.5 MG/~~HR~~ X 6 ~~HR~~ = 63 MG
63 ~~MG~~ / 50 ~~MG~~/ML = 1.26 ML LASIX

DILUTION:

1 ML/~~HR~~ X 6 ~~HR~~ = 6 ML TOTAL VOLUME
6 ML – 1.26 ML LASIX = 4.74 ML 0.9% NaCl = FLUID = X

Alright now we're doing some real work! Next up is the Fentanyl CRI. There will be multiple Fentanyl CRI's because I am going to show you some different ways this drug can be calculated and delivered. We also have straight and dilute Fentanyl CRI's so those will be reviewed in depth. Don't get overwhelmed! You're going to do just fine. Remember this drug is typically in micrograms not milligrams.

FENTANYL CRI (STRAIGHT – MCG/KG/HR)

LIGHT SENSITIVE

ORDER: 3 MCG/KG/HR
WEIGHT: 3.6 KG
RATE: X
TIME: 12 HR
CONC.: 50 MCG/ML

MCG/KG/HR:

3 MCG/KG/HR X 3.6 KG = 10.8 MCG/HR
10.8 MCG/HR X 12 HR = 129.6 MCG
129.6 MCG / 50 MCG/ML = 2.592 ML FENTANYL
2.592 ML / 12 HR = 0.216 ML/HR = RATE

Also if you ever need to convert MCG to MG:

$$\frac{3\ \text{MCG}}{1000\ \text{MCG}/\text{MG}} = 0.003\ \text{MG ORDER} \qquad \frac{50\ \text{MCG}}{1000\ \text{MCG}/\text{MG}} = 0.05\ \text{MG CONC}$$

MG/KG/HR:

0.003 MG/KG/HR X 3.6 KG = 0.0108 MG/HR
0.0108 MG/HR X 12 HR = 0.1296 MG
0.1296 MG / 0.05 MG/ML = 2.592 ML FENTANYL
2.592 ML / 12 HR = 0.216 ML/HR = RATE

See, not too terrible, right?

Now we will work with diluted Fentanyl CRI's before moving dosages up and down. There will be a simple method of how to calculate Fentanyl into a CRI on a syringe pump and then adding Fentanyl to a fluid bag and then and how to adjust dosages up and down from there. There's a little bit more work into those so we'll move from the easy to the more advanced stuff, okay? You're doing great!

FENTANYL CRI (DILUTE – MCG/KG/HR)

LIGHT SENSITIVE

ORDER: 4 MCG/KG/HR
WEIGHT: 6 KG
RATE: RUN AT 4 ML/HR
FLUID: X
TIME: 12 HR
CONC.: 50 MCG/ML

CALCULATE YOUR CRI:

4 MCG/~~KG~~/HR X 6 ~~KG~~ = 24 MCG/HR
24 MG/~~HR~~ X 12 ~~HR~~ = 288 MCG
288 ~~MCG~~ / 50 ~~MCG~~/ML = 5.76 ML FENTANYL

DILUTION:

4 ML/~~HR~~ X 12 ~~HR~~ = 48 ML
48 ML – 5.76 ML = 42.24 ML 0.9% NaCl = FLUIDS = X

INSTRUCTIONS:

1. DRAW UP 5.76 ML FENTANYL IN A SYRINGE
2. DRAW UP 42.24 ML DILUENT IN A SYRINGE
3. ADD SYRINGES TOGETHER = 48 ML
4. SET YOUR SYRINGE PUMP RATE TO 4 ML/HR AND YOUR VTBI TO 48 ML AND YOUR TIME SHOULD BE 12 HR AS A CHECK.

FENTANYL CRI (DILUTE – MCG/KG/HR IN FLUID BAG)

LIGHT SENSITIVE

ORDER: 5 MCG/KG/HR
WEIGHT: 20 KG
RATE: 5 ML/KG/HR = X
FLUID: 1L = 1000 ML
TIME: Y
CONC.: 50 MCG/ML

CALCULATE YOUR RATE AND FLUID BAG TIME FIRST:

5 ML/~~KG~~/HR X 20 KG = 100 ML/HR = RATE = X
1000 ~~ML~~ / 100 ~~ML~~/HR = 10 HR = TIME = Y

THEN CALCULATE YOUR FENTANYL CRI:

5 MCG/~~KG~~/HR X 20 ~~KG~~ = 100 MCG/HR
100 MCG/~~HR~~ X 10 ~~HR~~ = 1000 MCG
1000 ~~MCG~~ / 50 ~~MCG~~/ML = 20 ML FENTANYL

INSTRUCTIONS:

1. REMOVE 20ML OF FLUID FROM YOUR FLUID BAG
2. ADD 20ML OF FENTANYL TO YOUR FLUID BAG
3. MIX WELL
4. SET YOUR IV PUMP RATE TO 100 ML/HR AND YOUR VTBI TO 999 OR 1000 AND YOUR TIME SHOULD BE 9.99 OR 10 HRS AS A CHECK.

FENTANYL CRI (STRAIGHT - MOVING MCG UP)

LIGHT SENSITIVE

ORDER: INCREASE FROM 3 MCG/KG/HR TO 4 MCG/KG/HR
WEIGHT: 25 KG
RATE: X
TIME: 12 HR
CONC.: 50 MCG/ML

FIRST, FIND 3 MCG/KG/HR:

3 MCG/~~KG~~/HR X 25 ~~KG~~ = 75 MCG/HR
75 MCG/~~HR~~ X 12 ~~HR~~ = 900 MCG
900 ~~MCG~~ / 50 ~~MCG~~/ML = 18 ML FENTANYL DRUG VOLUME
18 ML / 12 HR = 1.5 ML/HR = CURRENT RATE

THEN, FIND 1 MCG/KG/HR:

1 MCG/~~KG~~/HR X 25 ~~KG~~ = 25 MCG/HR
25 ~~MCG~~/HR / 50 ~~MCG~~/ML = 0.5 ML/HR = RATE OF CHANGE

THEN ADD YOUR RATE OF CHANGE AND YOUR CURRENT RATE
TOGETHER FOR YOUR NEW RATE WHICH IS EQUAL TO 4
MCG/KG/HR:

1.5 ML/HR + 0.5 ML/HR = 2 ML/HR FENTANYL = RATE = X

Make sure your new label states: FENTANYL - STRAIGHT
4 MCG/KG/HR = 2 ML/HR

FENTANYL CRI (STRAIGHT – MOVING MCG DOWN)

LIGHT SENSITIVE

ORDER: DECREASE FROM 4 MCG/KG/HR TO 3 MCG/KG/HR
WEIGHT: 25 KG
RATE: X
TIME: 6 HR
CONC.: 50 MCG/ML

FIRST, FIND 4 MCG/KG/HR:

4 MCG/~~KG~~/HR X 25 ~~KG~~ = 100 MCG/HR
100 MCG/~~HR~~ X 6 ~~HR~~ = 600 MCG
600 ~~MCG~~ / 50 ~~MCG~~/ML = 12 ML FENTANYL DRUG VOLUME
12 ML / 6 HR = 2 ML/HR = CURRENT RATE

THEN, FIND 1 MCG/KG/HR AND THE RATE OF CHANGE:

1 MCG/~~KG~~/HR X 25 ~~KG~~ = 25 MCG/HR
25 ~~MCG~~/HR / 50 ~~MCG~~/ML = 0.5 ML/HR = RATE OF CHANGE

THEN SUBTRACT YOUR CURRENT RATE AND YOUR RATE OF CHANGE FOR YOUR NEW RATE WHICH IS EQUAL TO 3 MCG/KG/HR:

2 ML/HR - 0.5 ML/HR = 1.5 ML/HR FENTANYL = RATE = X

Make sure your new label states: FENTANYL - STRAIGHT
3 MCG/KG/HR = 1.5 ML/HR

Congratulations! You've just mastered Midazolam, Diazepam, Furosemide, and Fentanyl CRI's! Take a moment to celebrate! This is a big step as Fentanyl CRI's and dilutions can be challenging.

Now we'll work on creating 1 ML/HR and 2 ML/HR dilutions!

CREATING A 1 ML/HR DILUTION

This method can be used for any drug that equals <1 ML/HR to be run at 1 ML/HR.

DRUG: FENTANYL CRI (STRAIGHT TO DILUTE)
RATE: 0.36 ML/HR, RUN AT 1 ML/HR
TIME: 12 HR

0.36 ML/HR X 12 HR = 4.32 ML FENTANYL

1 ML/HR X 12 HR = 12 ML TOTAL VOLUME

12 ML – 4.32 ML = 7.68 ML DILUENT

7.68 ML DILUENT + 4.32 ML FENTANYL = 12 ML TOTAL VOLUME

CREATING A 2 ML/HR DILUTION

This method can be used for an extension set that is not a microbore

DRUG: FENTANYL CRI (STRAIGHT TO DILUTE)
RATE: 0.36 ML/HR, RUN AT 2 ML/HR
TIME: 12 HR

0.36 ML/HR X 12 HR = 4.32 ML FENTANYL

2 ML/HR X 12 HR = 24 ML TOTAL VOLUME

24 ML – 4.32 ML = 19.68 ML DILUENT

19.68 ML DILUENT + 4.32 ML FENTANYL = 24 ML TOTAL VOLUME

Now we are going to work on Dobutamine, Dopamine, Lidocaine, Ketamine and Metoclopramide! These are typically in MCG/KG/MIN or MG/KG/DAY so there can be some additional steps in converting minutes to hours so that you can get your rate in ML/HR and converting micrograms to milligrams so you can divide by your concentration.

DOBUTAMINE CRI (DILUTE – MCG/KG/MIN – ON SYRINGE PUMP)

ORDER: 10 MCG/KG/MIN
WEIGHT: 31 KG
RATE: RUN AT 10 ML/HR
FLUID: 60 ML 0.9% NaCl
TIME: X
CONC.: 12.5 MG/ML

CALCULATE YOUR FLUID TIME:

FLUID / RATE = TIME
60 ~~ML~~ / 10 ~~ML~~/HR = 6 HR

CALCULATE YOUR CRI:

10 MCG/~~KG~~/MIN X 31 ~~KG~~ = 310 MCG/MIN
310 MCG/~~MIN~~ X 60 ~~MIN~~/HR = 18,600 MCG/HR
18,600 ~~MCG~~/HR / 1000 ~~MCG~~/MG = 18.6 MG/HR
18.6 MG/~~HR~~ X 6 ~~HR~~ = 111.6 MG
111.6 ~~MG~~ / 12.5 ~~MG~~/ML = 8.9 ML DOBUTAMINE

CALCULATE YOUR DILUTION:

60 ML 0.9% NaCl – 8.9 ML DOBUTAMINE = 51.1 ML 0.9% NaCl

DOBUTAMINE CRI (STRAIGHT - MCG/KG/MIN INCREASING AND DECREASING RATE)

ORDER: 10 MCG/KG/MIN CHANGED TO 12 MCG/KG/MIN
WEIGHT: 31 KG
RATE: X
TIME: 6 HR
CONC.: 12.5 MG/ML

CALCULATE YOUR 10 MCG/KG/MIN CRI:

10 MCG/~~KG~~/MIN X 31 ~~KG~~ = 310 MCG/MIN
310 MCG/~~MIN~~ X 60 ~~MIN~~/HR = 18,600 MCG/HR
18,600 ~~MCG~~/HR / 1000 ~~MCG~~/MG = 18.6 MG/HR
18.6 MG/~~HR~~ X 6 ~~HR~~ = 111.6 MG
111.6 ~~MG~~ / 12.5 ~~MG~~/ML = 8.93 ML DOBUTAMINE

CALCULATE YOUR RATE:

18.6 ~~MG~~/HR / 12.5 ~~MG~~/ML = 1.488 ML/HR = 1.49 ML/HR AT 10 MCG/KG/MIN

CALCULATE 1 MCG/KG/MIN TO FIND CHANGE OF RATE PER 1 MCG/KG/MIN:

1 MCG/~~KG~~/MIN X 31 ~~KG~~ = 31 MCG/MIN
31 MCG/~~MIN~~ X 60 ~~MIN~~/HR = 1860 MCG/HR
1860 ~~MCG~~/HR / 1000 ~~MCG~~/MG = 1.86 MG/HR
1.86 ~~MG~~/HR / 12.5 ~~MG~~/ML = 0.1488 ML/HR = 0.15 ML/HR ROUNDED PER 1 MCG/KG/MIN

CALCULATE CHANGE OF RATE AND ORDER TO 12 MCG/KG/MIN:

WE NEED TO GO UP 2 MCG/KG/MIN, CHANGE OF RATE IS 0.15 ML/HR PER 1 MCG/KG/MIN:

0.15 ML/HR X 2 = 0.3 ML/HR
1.49 ML/HR + 0.3 ML/HR = 1.79 ML/HR = 1.8 ML/HR @ 12 MCG/KG/MIN

WE CAN ALSO MOVE DOWN AS NEEDED:

ORDER: 12 MCG/KG/MIN CHANGED TO 9 MCG/KG/MIN
WEIGHT: 31 KG
RATE: X
TIME: 6 HR
CONC.: 12.5 MG/ML

CHANGE ORDER FROM 12 MCG/KG/MIN DOWN TO 9 MCG/KG/MIN:

12 MCG/KG/HR = 1.79 ML/HR
RATE OF CHANGE = 0.15 ML/HR PER 1 MCG/KG/MIN

12 MCG/KG/MIN – 9 MCG/KG/MIN = 3 MCG/KG/MIN
0.15 ML/HR X 3 = 0.45 ML/HR
1.79 ML/HR – 0.45 ML/HR = 1.34 ML/HR @ 9 MCG/KG/MIN

DOPAMINE CRI (DILUTE - MCG/KG/MIN - ON SYRINGE PUMP)

LIGHT SENSITIVE

ORDER: 5 MCG/KG/MIN
WEIGHT: 15 KG
RATE: 5 ML/HR
FLUID: 60 ML 0.9% NaCl
TIME: X
CONC.: 40 MG/ML

CALCULATE YOUR FLUID TIME FIRST:

FLUIDS / RATE = TIME
60 ~~ML~~ / 5 ~~ML~~/HR = 12 HR

CALCULATE YOUR CRI:

5 MCG/~~KG~~/MIN X 15 ~~KG~~ = 75 MCG/MIN
75 MCG/~~MIN~~ X 60 ~~MIN~~/HR = 4500 MCG/HR
4500 MCG/~~HR~~ X 12 ~~HR~~ = 54,000 MCG
54,000 ~~MCG~~ / 1000 ~~MCG~~/MG = 54 MG
54 ~~MG~~ / 40 ~~MG~~/ML = 1.35 ML DOPAMINE

CALCULATE YOUR DILUTION:

60 ML – 1.35 ML DOPAMINE = 58.65 ML 0.9% NaCl

LIDOCAINE CRI (STRAIGHT – MCG/KG/MIN – SYRINGE PUMP)

LIGHT SENSITIVE

ORDER: 50 MCG/KG/MIN
WEIGHT: 38 KG
RATE: X
TIME: 10 HR
CONC.: 20 MG/ML

CALCULATE YOUR CRI:

50 MCG/~~KG~~/MIN X 38 ~~KG~~ = 1900 MCG/MIN

1900 MCG/~~MIN~~ X 60 ~~MIN~~/HR = 114,000 MCG/HR

114,000 ~~MCG~~/HR / 1000 ~~MCG~~/MG = 114 MG/HR

114 MG/~~HR~~ X 10 ~~HR~~ = 1140 MG

1140 ~~MG~~/HR / 20 ~~MG~~/ML = 57 ML LIDOCAINE TOTAL VOLUME

CALCULATE YOUR RATE:

TOTAL VOLUME / TIME = RATE
57 ML LIDOCAINE / 10 HR = 5.7 ML/HR = RATE = X

LIDOCAINE CRI (DILUTE - MCG/KG/MIN - FLUID BAG)

LIGHT SENSITIVE

ORDER: 60 MCG/KG/MIN
WEIGHT: 15 KG
RATE: 1XM @ 60 ML/KG/DAY
FLUID: 1L OF NORM-R
TIME: X
CONC.: 20 MG/ML

CALCULATE YOUR MAINTENANCE RATE FIRST:

60 ML/~~KG~~/DAY X 15 ~~KG~~ = 900 ML/DAY
900 ML/~~DAY~~ / 24 HR/~~DAY~~ = 37.5 ML/HR = RATE

CALCULATE YOUR FLUID BAG TIME:

1L = 1000 ~~ML~~ / 37.5 ~~ML~~/HR = 26.67 HR = TIME = X

CALCULATE YOUR CRI:

60 MCG/~~KG~~/MIN X 15 ~~KG~~ = 900 MCG/MIN
900 MCG/~~MIN~~ X 60 ~~MIN~~/HR = 54,000 MCG/HR
54,000 MCG/~~HR~~ X 26.67 ~~HR~~ = 1,440,000 MCG
1,440,000 ~~MCG~~ / 1000 ~~MCG~~/MG = 1,440 MG
1,440 ~~MG~~ / 20 ~~MG~~/ML = 72 ML

CALCULATE YOUR DILUTION:

1000 ML – 72 ML LIDOCAINE = 928 ML OF FLUID

PULL 72 ML OF FLUID FROM YOUR FLUID BAG FIRST, THEN ADD 72 ML LIDOCAINE AND MIX WELL.

KETAMINE CRI (DILUTE - MCG/KG/MIN CONVERTED TO MG/KG/HR)

LIGHT SENSITIVE

ORDER: 2 MCG/KG/MIN
WEIGHT: 20 KG
RATE: RUN AT 1 ML/HR
TIME: 20 HR
FLUID: X
CONC.: 100 MG/ML

LOADING DOSAGE: 500 MCG/KG = 0.5 MG/KG IV
CRI DOSAGE RANGE: 2 MCG/KG/MIN - 10 MCG/KG/MIN = 0.1 MG/KG/HR - 0.6 MG/KG/HR

LOADING DOSE IN MCG/KG:

500 MCG/~~KG~~ X 20 ~~KG~~ = 10,000 MCG
10,000 ~~MCG~~ / 1000 ~~MCG~~/MG = 10 MG
10 ~~MG~~ / 100 ~~MG~~/ML = 0.1 ML KETAMINE IV BOLUS

MCG/KG/MIN CRI:

2 MCG/~~KG~~/MIN X 20 ~~KG~~ = 40 MCG/MIN
40 MCG/~~MIN~~ X 60 ~~MIN~~/HR = 2400 MCG/HR
2400 ~~MCG~~/HR / 1000 ~~MCG~~/MG = 2.4 MG/HR
2.4 MG/~~HR~~ X 20 ~~HR~~ = 48 MG
48 ~~MG~~ / 100 ~~MG~~/ML = 0.48 ML KETAMINE

DILUTION:

1 ML/HR X 20 HR = 20 ML TOTAL VOLUME
20 ML – 0.48 ML = 19.52 ML DILUENT = FLUIDS = X

OR CONVERT MCG/KG/MIN TO MG/KG/HR:

2 ~~MCG~~/KG/MIN / 1000 ~~MCG~~/MG = 0.002 MG/KG/MIN
0.002 MG/KG/~~MIN~~ X 60 ~~MIN~~/HR = 0.12 MG/KG/HR

LOADING DOSE IN MG/KG:

0.5 MG/~~KG~~ X 20 ~~KG~~ = 10 MG
10 ~~MG~~ / 100 ~~MG~~/ML = 0.1 ML KETAMINE IV BOLUS

MG/KG/HR CRI:

0.12 MG/~~KG~~/HR X 20 ~~KG~~ = 2.4 MG/HR
2.4 MG/~~HR~~ X 20 ~~HR~~ = 48 MG
48 ~~MG~~ / 100 ~~MG~~/ML = 0.48 ML KETAMINE

DILUTION:

1 ML/~~HR~~ X 20 ~~HR~~ = 20 ML
20 ML – 0.48 ML = 19.52 ML DILUENT = FLUIDS = X

METOCLOPRAMIDE CRI (DILUTE – MG/KG/DAY – CALCULATION OF FLUID LEFT IN BAG)

LIGHT SENSITIVE

ORDER: 2 MG/KG/DAY
WEIGHT: 4.72 KG
RATE: 2XM @ 120 ML/KG/DAY
FLUID: 500 ML LEFT OF 1L OF NORM-R
TIME: X
CONC.: 5 MG/ML

CALCULATE RATE AND FLUID BAG TIME:

120 ML/~~KG~~/DAY X 4.72 ~~KG~~ = 566.4 ML/DAY
566.4 ML/~~DAY~~ / 24 HR/~~DAY~~ = 23.6 ML/HR = RATE

500 ~~ML~~ / 23.6 ~~ML~~/HR = 21.18 HR = TIME = X

CALCULATE YOUR CRI:

2 MG/~~KG~~/DAY X 4.72 ~~KG~~ = 9.44 MG/DAY
9.44 MG/~~DAY~~ / 24 HR/~~DAY~~ = 0.393 MG/HR
0.393 MG/~~HR~~ X 21.18 ~~HR~~ = 8.32 MG
8.32 ~~MG~~ / 5 ~~MG~~/ML = 1.66 ML METOCLOPRAMIDE TO 500 ML N/R

METOCLOPRAMIDE CRI (DILUTE - MG/KG/DAY - CALCULATION OF 1L)
LIGHT SENSITIVE

ORDER: 2 MG/KG/DAY
WEIGHT: 18 KG
RATE: 1XM @ 60 ML/KG/DAY
FLUID: 1L OF PLA
TIME: X
CONC.: 5 MG/ML

CALCULATE YOUR MAINTENANCE FLUID RATE AND FLUID BAG TIME FIRST:

60 ML/~~KG~~/DAY X 18 ~~KG~~ = 1080 ML/DAY
1080 ML/~~DAY~~ / 24 HR/~~DAY~~ = 45 ML/HR = RATE

1L = 1000 ~~ML~~ / 45 ~~ML~~/HR = 22.2 HR = TIME = X

CALCULATE YOUR CRI:

2 MG/~~KG~~/DAY X 18 ~~KG~~ = 36 MG/DAY
36 MG/~~DAY~~ / 24 HR/~~DAY~~ = 1.5 MG/HR
1.5 MG/~~HR~~ X 22.2 ~~HR~~ = 33.3 MG
33.3 ~~MG~~ / 5 ~~MG~~/ML = 6.66 ML METOCLOPRAMIDE TO 1L PLA

METOCLOPRAMIDE CRI (MG/KG/DAY - CALCULATION FOR SYRINGE)

LIGHT SENSITIVE

ORDER: 2 MG/KG/DAY
WEIGHT: 18 KG
RATE: RUN AT 2 ML/HR
FLUID: 60 ML 0.9% NaCl
TIME: X
CONC.: 5 MG/ML

CALCULATE YOUR TIME:

FLUID / RATE = TIME
60 ML / 2 ML/HR = 30 HR

CALCULATE YOUR CRI:

2 MG/KG/DAY X 18 KG = 36 MG/DAY
36 MG/DAY / 24 HRS/DAY = 1.5 MG/HR
1.5 MG/HR X 30 HR = 45 MG
45 MG / 5 MG/ML = 9 ML METOCLOPRAMIDE

DILUTION:
60 ML – 9 ML METOCLOPRAMIDE = 51 ML 0.9% NaCl

Great job! Now we're going to work on FLK's, HLK's, and MLK's in fluid bags and running them at surgical rates in ML/KG/HR. Don't worry, we'll work on one drug at a time and you'll be a pro in no time!

FLK CRI (ML/KG/HR)
FENTANYL/LIDOCAINE/KETAMINE, LIGHT SENSITIVE

STANDARD ORDER: 1 ML/KG/HR
INTRA-OP ORDER: 2 ML/KG/HR
WEIGHT: 15 KG
FLUID: 1L BAG 0.09% NaCl/NORM-R/LRS/PLASMALYTE

CALCULATE YOUR RATE & FLUID BAG TIME FIRST:
2 ML/~~KG~~/HR X 15 ~~KG~~ = 30 ML/HR = RATE
1000 ~~ML~~ / 30 ~~ML~~/HR = 33.3 HR = FLUID BAG TIME

F: 50 MCG/ML = 0.05 MG/ML CONC.
  LOADING DOSE RANGE: 0.5 MCG/KG – 3 MCG/KG =
  0.0005 MG/KG – 0.003 MG/KG IV BOLUS
  CRI DOSAGE RANGE: 0.5 MCG/KG/HR – 3 MCG/KG/HR =
  0.0005 MG/KG/HR – 0.003 MG/KG/HR

  LOADING DOSAGE: 2 MCG/KG = 0.002 MG/KG
  CRI DOSAGE: 2 MCG/KG/HR = 0.002 MG/KG/HR

  LOADING DOSE:
  2 MCG/~~KG~~ X 15 ~~KG~~ = 30 MCG
  30 ~~MCG~~ / 50 ~~MCG~~/ML = 0.6 ML IV FENTANYL BOLUS

  CRI:
  2 MCG/~~KG~~/HR X 15 ~~KG~~ = 30 MCG/HR
  30 MCG/~~HR~~ X 33.3 ~~HR~~ = 999 MCG
  999 ~~MCG~~ / 50 ~~MCG~~/ML = 19.98 ML = 20 ML FENTANYL

L: 20 MG/ML CONC.

LOADING DOSE RANGE: 2000 MCG/KG = 2 MG/KG IV BOLUS
CRI DOSAGE RANGE: 16.67 MCG/KG/MIN – 33.3 MCG/KG/MIN = 1 MG/KG/HR – 2 MG/KG/HR

LOADING DOSAGE: 2000 MCG/KG = 2 MG/KG
CRI DOSAGE: 16.67 MCG/KG/MIN = 1 MG/KG/HR

LOADING DOSE:
2 MG/~~KG~~ X 15 ~~KG~~ = 30 MG
30 ~~MG~~ / 20 ~~MG~~/ML = 1.5 ML IV LIDOCAINE BOLUS

CRI:
1 MG/~~KG~~/HR X 15 ~~KG~~ = 15 MG/HR
15 MG/~~HR~~ X 33.3 ~~HR~~ = 499.5 MG
499.5 ~~MG~~ / 20 ~~MG~~/ML = 24.975 ML = 25 ML LIDOCAINE

K: 100 MG/ML CONC.

LOADING DOSE RANGE: 500 MCG/KG – 2000 MCG/KG = 0.5 MG/KG – 2 MG/KG IV BOLUS
CRI DOSAGE RANGE: 2 MCG/KG/MIN – 10 MCG/KG/MIN = 0.12 MG/KG/HR – 0.6 MG/KG/HR

LOADING DOSAGE: 500 MCG/KG = 0.5 MG/KG
CRI DOSAGE: 2.5 MCG/KG/MIN = 0.15 MG/KG/HR

LOADING DOSE:
0.5 MG/~~KG~~ X 15 ~~KG~~ = 7.5 MG
7.5 ~~MG~~ / 100 ~~MG~~/ML = 0.075 ML IV KETAMINE BOLUS

CRI:

0.15 MG/~~KG~~/HR X 15 ~~KG~~ = 2.25 MG/HR

2.25 MG/~~HR~~ X 33.3 ~~HR~~ = 74.925 MG

74.925 ~~MG~~ / 100 ~~MG~~/ML = 0.749 ML = 0.75 ML KETAMINE

F: 20 ML

L: 25 ML

K: 0.75 ML

20 ML FENTANYL + 25 ML LIDOCAINE + 0.75 ML KETAMINE = 45.75 ML

INSTRUCTIONS: REMOVE 45.75 ML FROM 1000 ML BAG FIRST AND REPLACE WITH ALL THREE DRUGS WHICH IS EQUIVALENT TO 45.75 ML

MLK CRI (ML/KG/HR)
MORPHINE/LIDOCAINE/KETAMINE, LIGHT SENSITIVE

ORDER: 2 ML/KG/HR
WEIGHT: 15 KG
FLUID: 1L BAG 0.09% NaCl/NORM-R/LRS/PLASMALYTE

CALCULATE YOUR RATE AND FLUID BAG TIME FIRST:
2 ML/~~KG~~/HR X 15 ~~KG~~ = 30 ML/HR = RATE
1L = 1000 ~~ML~~ / 30 ~~ML~~/HR = 33.3 HR = FLUID BAG TIME

M: 15 MG/ML CONC
   LOADING DOSE RANGE: 200 MCG/KG – 400 MCG/KG =
   0.2 MG/KG – 0.4 MG/KG IV BOLUS
   CRI DOSAGE RANGE: 1.67 MCG/KG/MIN – 6.67 MCG/KG/MIN =
   0.1 MG/KG/HR – 0.4 MG/KG/HR

   LOADING DOSAGE: 200 MCG/KG = 0.2 MG/KG
   CRI DOSAGE: 2.5 MCG/KG/MIN = 0.15 MG/KG/HR

   LOADING DOSE:
   0.2 MG/~~KG~~ X 15 ~~KG~~ = 3 MG
   3 ~~MG~~ / 15 ~~MG~~/ML = 0.2 ML IV MORPHINE BOLUS

   CRI:
   0.15 MG/~~KG~~/HR X 15 ~~KG~~ = 2.25 MG/HR
   2.25 MG/~~HR~~ X 33.3 ~~HR~~ = 74.925 MG
   74.925 ~~MG~~ / 15 ~~MG~~/ML = 4.995 ML = 5 ML MORPHINE

L: 20 MG/ML CONC.

LOADING DOSE RANGE: 2000 MCG/KG = 2 MG/KG IV BOLUS
CRI DOSAGE RANGE: 16.67 MCG/KG/MIN – 33.3 MCG/KG/MIN = 1 MG/KG/HR – 2 MG/KG/HR

LOADING DOSAGE: 2000 MCG/KG = 2 MG/KG
CRI DOSAGE: 25 MCG/KG/MIN = 1.5 MG/KG/HR

LOADING DOSE:
2 MG/~~KG~~ X 15 ~~KG~~ = 30 MG
30 ~~MG~~ / 20 ~~MG~~/ML = 1.5 ML IV LIDOCAINE BOLUS

CRI:
1.5 MG/~~KG~~/HR X 15 ~~KG~~ = 22.5 MG/HR
22.5 MG/~~HR~~ X 33.3 ~~HR~~ = 749.25 MG
749.25 ~~MG~~ / 20 ~~MG~~/ML = 37.46 ML = 37.5 ML LIDOCAINE

K: 100 MG/ML CONC.

LOADING DOSE RANGE: 500 MCG/KG – 2000 MCG/KG = 0.5 MG/KG – 2 MG/KG IV BOLUS
CRI DOSAGE RANGE: 2 MCG/KG/MIN – 10 MCG/KG/MIN = 0.12 MG/KG/HR – 0.6 MG/KG/HR

LOADING DOSAGE: 500 MCG/KG = 0.5 MG/KG
CRI DOSAGE: 2.5 MCG/KG/MIN = 0.15 MG/KG/HR

LOADING DOSE:
0.5 MG/~~KG~~ X 15 ~~KG~~ = 7.5 MG
7.5 ~~MG~~ / 100 ~~MG~~/ML = 0.075 ML IV KETAMINE BOLUS

CRI:

0.15 MG/~~KG~~/HR X 15 ~~KG~~ = 2.25 MG/HR

2.25 MG/~~HR~~ X 33.3 ~~HR~~ = 74.925 MG

74.925 ~~MG~~ / 100 ~~MG~~/ML = 0.749 ML = 0.75 ML KETAMINE

M: 5 ML
L: 37.5 ML
K: 0.75 ML

5 ML MORPHINE + 37.5 ML LIDOCAINE + 0.75 ML KETAMINE = 43.25 ML

INSTRUCTIONS: REMOVE 43.25 ML FROM 1L BAG FIRST AND REPLACE WITH ALL THREE DRUGS WHICH IS EQUIVALENT TO 43.25 ML

HLK CRI (ML/KG/HR)
HYDROMORPHONE/LIDOCAINE/KETAMINE, LIGHT SENSITIVE

ORDER: 1 ML/KG/HR
WEIGHT: 15 KG
FLUID: 1L BAG 0.09% NaCl/NORM-R/LRS/PLASMALYTE

CALCULATE YOUR RATE AND FLUID BAG TIME FIRST:
1 ML/~~KG~~/HR X 15 ~~KG~~ = 15 ML/HR
1L = 1000 ~~ML~~ / 15 ~~ML~~/HR = 66.67 HR

H: 2 MG/ML CONC
    LOADING DOSE RANGE: 30 MCG/KG – 75 MCG/KG =
    0.03 MG/KG – 0.075 MG/KG IV BOLUS
    CRI DOSAGE RANGE: 0.5 MCG/KG/MIN – 0.83 MCG/KG/MIN =
    0.03 MG/KG/HR – 0.05 MG/KG/HR

    LOADING DOSAGE: 30 MCG/KG = 0.03 MG/KG
    CRI DOSAGE: 0.5 MCG/KG/MIN = 0.03 MG/KG/HR

    LOADING DOSE:
    0.03 MG/~~KG~~ X 15 ~~KG~~ = 0.45 MG
    0.45 ~~MG~~ / 2 ~~MG~~/ML = 0.225 ML = 0.23 ML IV HYDROMORPHONE
    BOLUS

    CRI:
    0.03 MG/~~KG~~/HR X 15 ~~KG~~ = 0.45 MG/HR
    0.45 MG/~~HR~~ X 66.67 ~~HR~~ = 30.0015 MG
    30.0015 ~~MG~~ / 2 ~~MG~~/ML = 15 ML HYDROMORPHONE

L: 20 MG/ML CONC.
   LOADING DOSE RANGE: 2000 MCG/KG = 2 MG/KG IV BOLUS
   CRI DOSAGE RANGE: 16.67 MCG/KG/MIN – 33.3 MCG/KG/MIN =
   1 MG/KG/HR – 2 MG/KG/HR

   LOADING DOSAGE: 2000 MCG/KG = 2 MG/KG
   CRI DOSAGE: 25 MCG/KG/MIN = 1.5 MG/KG/HR

   LOADING DOSE:
   2 MG/~~KG~~ X 15 ~~KG~~ = 30 MG
   30 ~~MG~~ / 20 ~~MG~~/ML = 1.5 ML IV LIDOCAINE BOLUS

   CRI:
   1.5 MG/~~KG~~/HR X 15 ~~KG~~ = 22.5 MG/HR
   22.5 MG/~~HR~~ X 66.67 ~~HR~~ = 1500.075 MG
   1500.075 ~~MG~~ / 20 ~~MG~~/ML = 75 ML LIDOCAINE

K: 100 MG/ML CONC
   LOADING DOSE RANGE: 500 MCG/KG – 2000 MCG/KG =
   0.5 MG/KG – 2 MG/KG IV BOLUS
   CRI DOSAGE RANGE: 2 MCG/KG/MIN – 10 MCG/KG/MIN =
   0.12 MG/KG/HR – 0.6 MG/KG/HR

   LOADING DOSAGE: 500 MCG/KG = 0.5 MG/KG
   CRI DOSAGE: 2 MCG/KG/MIN = 0.12 MG/KG/HR

   LOADING DOSE:
   0.5 MG/~~KG~~ X 15 ~~KG~~ = 7.5 MG
   7.5 ~~MG~~ / 100 ~~MG~~/ML = 0.075 ML IV KETAMINE BOLUS

CRI:

0.12 MG/~~KG~~/HR X 15 ~~KG~~ = 1.8 MG/HR

1.8 MG/~~HR~~ X 66.67 ~~HR~~ = 120.006 MG

120.006 MG / 100 MG/ML = 1.2 ML KETAMINE

H: 15 ML
L: 75 ML
K: 1.2 ML

15 ML HYDROMORPHONE + 75 ML LIDOCAINE + 1.2 ML KETAMINE = 91.2 ML

INSTRUCTIONS: REMOVE 91.2 ML FROM 1L BAG FIRST AND REPLACE WITH ALL THREE DRUGS WHICH IS EQUIVALENT TO 91.2 ML

CHAPTER 8:
IV FLUID ADDITIVES

KCl CHART

20 mEq/L

ADD 2mEq/mL KCl	TO FLUID AMOUNT
30 ML	3000 ML
10 ML	1000 ML* IVF BAG
5 ML	500 ML
1 ML	100 ML* BURETROL
0.5 ML	50 ML

30 mEq/L

ADD 2mEq/mL KCl	TO FLUID AMOUNT
45 ML	3000 ML
15 ML	1000 ML* IVF BAG
7.5 ML	500 ML
1.5 ML	100 ML* BURETROL
0.75 ML	50 ML

KCl ADDED TO BURETROL

ORDER: 30 mEq/L
FLUID: 100 ML BURETROL
CONC: 2 mEq/ML

30 ~~mEq~~/L / 2 ~~mEq~~/ML = 15 ML/L
100 ~~ML~~ / 1000 ~~ML~~/L = 0.1 L
15 ML/~~L~~ X 0.1 ~~L~~ (% of 1L: 10% = 100 ML) = 1.5 ML KCl

1.5 ML OF KCl IS ADDED TO 100 ML OF FLUID FOR A 30 mEq/L
SOLUTION

*KCl is ALWAYS an IVF additive! DO NOT BOLUS!

KCl ADDED TO IV FLUID BAG TO INCREASE CONCENTRATION

ORDER: 20 mEq/L in 900 ML fluid bag, increase to 30 mEq/L
CONC.: 2 mEq/mL

1. 30 mEq/L
   <u>- 20 mEq/L</u>
   10 mEq/L

2. $\frac{10 \text{ mEq/L}}{2 \text{ mEq/ML}}$ = 5 ML/L

3. 900 ML / 1000 ML/L = 0.9 L

4. 5 ML/L x 0.9 L (% of bag left) (90% = 900 ML) = 4.5 ML KCl added to IVF bag to increase concentration from 20 mEq/L to 30 mEq/L.

*KCl is ALWAYS an IVF additive! DO NOT BOLUS!

KPHOS ADDED TO BURETROL – MMOL/KG/HR

CRI DOSAGE RANGE: 0.01-0.06 MMOL/KG/HR
ORDER: 0.01 MMOL/KG/HR
WEIGHT: 15 KG
RATE: 1XM = 60 ML/KG/DAY
FLUIDS: 0.9% NaCl IN BURETROL
DOSAGE: Y
TIME: 4 HOURS (RE-ASSESS q4-6H)
CONC: 3 MMOL/ML PHOS
      4.4 mEq/ML K

FLUID RATE AND VOLUME CALCULATION AT 1XM:

60 ML/~~KG~~/DAY X 15 ~~KG~~ = 900 ML/DAY
900 ML/~~DAY~~ / 24 HR/~~DAY~~ = 37.5 ML/HR = RATE = X
37.5 ML/~~HR~~ X 4 ~~HR~~ = 150 ML 0.9% NaCl IN BURETROL

KPHOS CRI CALCULATION:

0.01 MMOL/~~KG~~/HR X 15 ~~KG~~ = 0.15 MMOL/HR
0.15 MMOL/~~HR~~ X 4 ~~HR~~ = 0.6 MMOL
0.6 ~~MMOL~~ / 3 ~~MMOL~~/ML = 0.2 ML KPHOS

0.2 ML KPHOS is practically a negligible amount and is fine to add to a 150 ML buretrol.

*KPHOS is ALWAYS an IVF additive! DO NOT BOLUS!

KPHOS ADDED TO BURETROL – MEQ/L

ORDER: 40 mEq/L
WEIGHT: 15 KG
RATE: 1XM = 60 ML/KG DAY
FLUIDS: 0.9% NaCl IN BURETROL
DOSAGE: Y
TIME: 4 HOURS (RE-ASSESS q4-6H)
CONC: 3 MMOL/ML PHOS
      4.4 mEq/ML K

There are two ways to calculate this. Generally when an order is given in mEq's it's to calculate the Potassium component since this drug has more dire consequences if given too quickly or at too high of a concentration. Please ask your DVM which component of this drug they would like at 40 mEq/L.

1 MMOL/ML KPHOS = 1.8 mEq/ML KPHOS
3 MMOL/ML KPHOS = 5.4 mEq/ML KPHOS = CONC FOR PHOS COMPONENT IN mEq's

FLUID RATE AND VOLUME CALCULATION AT 1XM:

60 ML/KG/DAY X 15 KG = 900 ML/DAY
900 ML/DAY / 24 HR/DAY = 37.5 ML/HR = RATE = X
37.5 ML/HR X 4 HR = 150 ML 0.9% NaCl IN BURETROL

K COMPONENT CALCULATION IN mEq's:

40 mEq/L / 4.4 mEq/ML = 9.09 ML/L
9.09 ML/L X 0.15 L (15% of 1L = 150 ML) = 1.36 ML KPHOS

OR

PHOS COMPONENT CALCULATION IN mEq's:

40 ~~mEq~~/L / 5.4 ~~mEq~~/ML = 7.4 ML/L
7.4 ML/~~L~~ x 0.15 ~~L~~ (15% of 1L = 150 ML) = 1.11 ML KPHOS

HOW DO WE FIGURE OUT THE PERCENTAGE OF ML IN 1L?

150 ML / 1000 ML = 0.15 = 15%
60 ML / 1000 ML = 0.06 = 6%

MAGNESIUM 50% CONCENTRATION - DILUTE TO 20% (MEQ/KG/DAY)

5G PER 10 ML- 10 ML VIAL
CONC: 500 MG/ML
        4.06 mEq/ML

FOR SUSPECTED OR CONFIRMED HYPOMAGNESEMIA:

LOADING DOSE: 0.15 – 0.3 mEq/KG = 18.5 – 37 MG/KG DILUTED TO 20% CONCENTRATION AND GIVEN IV SLOW OVER 10-20 MINUTES
CRI: 0.75 – 1 mEq/KG/DAY = 92 – 123 MG/KG/DAY DILUTED TO 20% CONCENTRATION AND GIVEN IV OVER GIVEN TIME

FOR REFRACTORY VENTRICULAR DYSRHYTHMIAS:

0.15 – 0.3 mEq/KG IV ADMINISTERED SLOWLY OVER 10 MINUTES

MUST BE DILUTED TO 20% CONCENTRATION IN 0.9% NaCl, 0.45% NaCl or D5W

Not compatible with solutions containing 10% Lipid Emulsion (ILE's/Intralipids), Dobutamine, or solutions containing Calcium, Lactate, or Sodium Bicarbonate.

OVERDOSES: CALCIUM GLUCONATE FOR HYPERMAGNESEMIA

NORMAL MAGNESIUM REFERENCE RANGES

SPECIES	TOTAL Mg (MG/DL)	IONIZED Mg (MG/DL)
DOG	1.61-2.51*	1.03-1.36
CAT	1.70-2.99*	1.05-1.42

* = ANY VALUE <1.2 MG/DL NEEDS MAGNESIUM SUPPLEMENTATION

MAGNESIUM SUPPLEMENTATION IN PATIENTS WITH SERUM LEVELS <1.2 MG/DL:

<1.2 MG/DL = CRI AT 0.75 – 1 mEq/KG/DAY for 12 – 24 HOURS drop to 0.2 – 0.5 mEq/KG/DAY for additional 3 – 5 days. Check Magnesium serum levels every 6 – 12 hours. Daily dose can be given over 12-24 hours. Dosages should be reduced in animals with azotemia and/or renal insufficiency at a 50% – 75% reduction. Reduce daily dosages after the first day.

SCENARIO: IF A CANINE HAS A SERUM MAGNESIUM OF 1.1 MG/DL AND WE WANT TO CORRECT TO 2MG/DL WHAT DO WE NEED TO DO? WEIGHT = 27 KG, CREATININE = 1

$$\frac{\text{GOAL Mg} - \text{ACTUAL Mg}}{\text{CREATININE}} \quad \frac{2 \text{ MG/DL} - 1.1 \text{ MG/DL}}{1} = \frac{0.9 \text{ MG/DL}}{\text{TO CORRECT}}$$

SCENARIO: YOUR 27KG PATIENT NEEDS A 0.3 mEq/KG LOADING DOSE OF MAGNESIUM BEFORE INSTITUTING A 0.5 mEq/KG/DAY CRI FOR 12 HOURS. HOW MUCH MAGNESIUM SHOULD YOU GIVE AS A BOLUS? WHAT IS YOUR DILUTION? WHAT KIND OF DILUENTS ARE COMPATIBLE?

SOLUTION:

0.3 mEq/~~KG~~ X 27 ~~KG~~ = 8.1 mEq
8.1 ~~mEq~~ / 4.06 ~~mEq~~/ML = 1.99 ML 50% MAGNESIUM

DILUTION:

(C1)(V1)=(C2)(V2)
C1 = CONCENTRATION OF MEDICATION
V1 = VOLUME OF MEDICATION
C2 = FINAL CONCENTRATION OF MEDICATION
V2 = FINAL VOLUME OF MEDICATION
(C1)(V1)=(C2)(V2) = CALCULATE A NEW CONCENTRATION, SOLVE
FOR C2
(V2) – (V1) = CALCULATE HOW MUCH DILUENT TO ADD
(C1)(V1)=(C2)(V2) = CALCULATE A STARTING VOLUME, SOLVE FOR
V1

C1 = 50% MAGNESIUM
V1 = 1.99 ML
C2 = 20% MAGNESIUM SOLUTION
V2 = X

FIRST, (C1)(V1)=(C2)(V2)
(50%)(1.99 ML) = (20%)(V2)
    0.995 ML
(0.995 ML) = (20%)(V2)
   20%   20%

THEN, (V2) – (V1)
4.975 ML – 1.99 ML = 2.985 ML
2.99 ML DILUENT TO ADD TO MAGNESIUM TO MAKE A 20% CONCENTRATION

4.975 ML = (V2) = FINAL TOTAL
VOLUME OF MEDICATION

2 ML 50% MAGNESIUM + 3 ML DILUENT = 5 ML OF A 20%
SOLUTION TO BOLUS FOR LOADING DOSE

COMPATIBLE DILUENTS ARE: 0.9% NaCl, 0.45% NaCl, D5W

TO CALCULATE THE CRI, STATE YOUR KNOWN'S OR GIVEN'S:

ORDER: 0.5 mEq/KG/DAY
WEIGHT: 27 KG
RATE: X
FLUID: Y
TIME: 12 HOURS
CONC: 4.06mEq/ML; 50% DILUTED TO 20%

0.5 mEq/~~KG~~/DAY X 27 ~~KG~~ = 13.5 mEq/DAY
13.5 mEq/~~DAY~~ / 24 HR/~~DAY~~ = 0.5625 mEq/HR
0.5625 mEq/~~HR~~ x 12 ~~HR~~ = 6.75 mEq
6.75 ~~mEq~~ / 4.06 ~~mEq~~/ML = 1.66 ML MAGNESIUM

DILUTION:

C1 = 50% MAGNESIUM
V1 = 1.66 ML
C2 = 20% MAGNESIUM SOLUTION
V2 = X

FIRST, (C1)(V1)=(C2)(V2)
(50%)(1.66 ML) = (20%)(V2)
   0.83 ML
$\frac{(0.83 \text{ ML})}{20\%} = \frac{(20\%)(V2)}{20\%}$

THEN, (V2) – (V1)
4.15 ML – 1.66 ML = 2.49 ML
2.49 ML DILUENT TO ADD TO MAGNESIUM TO MAKE A 20% CONCENTRATION

4.15 ML = (V2) = FINAL TOTAL
VOLUME OF MEDICATION

1.7 ML MAGNESIUM + 2.5 ML DILUENT = 4.2 ML OF A 20% SOLUTION FOR CONSTANT RATE INFUSION OVER 12 HOURS.

RATE: 4.2 ML / 12 HR = 0.35 ML/HR ON SYRINGE PUMP

REASONS FOR DILUENT CHOICES:

0.9% NaCl – Na+ is WNL and fluid creep from sodium is not of much concern over the course of hospitalization.

0.45% NaCl – Na+ is high and/or fluid creep from sodium is a concern over the course of hospitalization.

D5W – Blood glucose is concurrently low or expected to drop out-of-range with ongoing hospitalization, or fluid creep from sodium is a concern over the course of hospitalization.

DEXTROSE CHART

2.5% DEXTROSE

ADD 50% DEXTROSE	TO FLUID AMOUNT
150 ML	3000 ML
50 ML	1000 ML* IVF BAG
25 ML	500 ML
5 ML	100 ML* BURETROL
0.5 ML	10 ML

5% DEXTROSE

ADD 50% DEXTROSE	TO FLUID AMOUNT
300 ML	3000 ML
100 ML	1000 ML* IVF BAG
50 ML	500 ML
10 ML	100 ML* BURETROL
1 ML	10 ML

5% DEXTROSE CALCULATION

250 ML OF FLUID   50% CONC. OF DEXTROSE

WANT 5% $250 \times 5(\%) = \dfrac{1250}{50(\%)} = 25$ ML

DEXTROSE CRI – DECREASING CONCENTRATION IN BURETROL

SCENARIO: DECREASE 7.5% DEXTROSE CRI TO 5% DEXTROSE WITH 68 ML LEFT IN BURETROL AT 7.5% CONCENTRATION.

SOLUTION:

$(C_1)(V_1)=(C_2)(V_2)$

C_1 = CONCENTRATION OF MEDICATION
V_1 = VOLUME OF MEDICATION
C_2 = FINAL CONCENTRATION OF MEDICATION
V_2 = FINAL VOLUME OF MEDICATION

$(C_1)(V_1)=(\underline{C_2})(V_2)$ = CALCULATE A NEW CONCENTRATION, SOLVE FOR C_2
$(V_2)-(V_1)$ = CALCULATE HOW MUCH DILUENT TO ADD
$(C_1)(\underline{V_1})=(C_2)(V_2)$ = CALCULATE A STARTING VOLUME, SOLVE FOR V_1

C_1 = 7.5% DEXTROSE
V_1 = 68 ML LEFT
C_2 = 5% DEXTROSE
V_2 = X

$(C_1)(V_1)=(C_2)(V_2)$
$\dfrac{(\underline{7.5\%})(68\ ML)}{5\%} = \dfrac{(\underline{5\%})(V_2)}{5\%}$
$(1.5\%)(68\ ML) = (V_2)$
$102\ ML = (V_2)$

THEN, $(V_2)-(V_1)$
102 ML – 68 ML = 34 ML
34 ML DILUENT TO ADD

DEXTROSE BOLUSES

DOSAGE: 0.5 – 1 ML/KG
DILUTE TO AT LEAST 10% (1:4) CONCENTRATION AND
GIVE IV SLOWLY OVER 5 MINUTES
ORDER: 1 ML/KG
WEIGHT: 20 KG
FLUID: 0.9% NaCl – DO NOT USE D5W
CONC: 50% = 500 MG/ML

1 ML/KG X 20 KG = 20 ML 50% DEXTROSE
50% / 10% = 5 (1:4 DILUTION, 5 TOTAL PARTS)
20 ML X 5 = 100 ML TOTAL VOLUME
100 ML – 20 ML = 80 ML DILUENT FOR 10% SOLUTION

CHECK:

10% DEXTROSE CALCULATION

100 ML OF FLUID   50% CONC. OF DEXTROSE
    WANT 10% $100 \times 10(\%) = \dfrac{1000}{50(\%)} = 20$ ML

CHAPTER 9:
VESICANTS & IRRITANTS

VESICANTS AND IRRITANTS

Vesicants are substances that can lead to cell death and tissue necrosis upon extravasation. **Extravasation** is the leakage of certain drugs (vesicants) out of a vein and into the surrounding tissue causing acute tissue injury that may be severe and lead to necrosis. **Irritants** are non-corrosive substances that cause a burning or an uncomfortable sensation upon infusion and cause a reversible inflammatory effect on living tissue by chemical action at the site of contact, according to O.S.H.A.

VESICANTS

COMMONLY USED IV MEDS
Gentamicin

Diazepam

Radiographic Contrast Media

Promethazine

VASOCOMPRESSIVE AGENTS
Dobutamine

Dopamine

Epinephrine

Norepinephrine

Vasopressin

CONCENTRATED ELECTROLYTE SOLUTIONS

Calcium Chloride

Calcium Gluconate 10%

Potassium Chloride 7.45%

Sodium Bicarbonate 4.2% and 8.4%

Sodium Chloride 10%

CYTOTOXIC/CHEMOTHERAPEUTIC AGENTS

Busulphan

Actinomycin-D

Danuorubicin

Doxorubicin

Epirubicin

Idarubicin

Mitomycin

Paclitaxel

Tresulfan

Vinblastine

Vincristine

Vinorelbine

HYPEROSMOLAR AGENTS

Total parenteral nutrition (TPN)

>10% Dextrose (25% Dextrose IS a vesicant, <u>do not</u> extravasate or just dilute to at least 10% concentration)

≥15% Mannitol

20% N-Acetylcysteine

IRRITANTS

Aminophylline

Potassium >60mEq/L

Penicillin

Amiodarone

Erythromycin

Metronidazole

Metoprolol

Phenobarbital

Propofol

CHAPTER 10:
INSULIN CRI , IV DRUG ADMINISTRATION, DEXDOMITOR CRI & PROPOFOL CRI

INSULIN CRI FOR CANINES AND FELINES

INSULIN CRI (CANINE)	INSULIN CRI (FELINE)
BINDS TO PLASTIC INSTRUCTIONS: 2.2 UNITS/KG OR 1 UNIT/LB REGULAR INSULIN PUT IN 250ML BAG OF 0.9% NaCl BLEED LINE OF 50ML'S BG'S q2-3h	BINDS TO PLASTIC INSTRUCTIONS: 1.1-2.2 UNITS/KG REGULAR INSULIN PUT IN 250ML BAG OF 0.9% NaCl BLEED LINE OF 50ML'S BG'S q2-3h

BG	IV FLUID COMPOSITION	INSULIN RATE
>350	0.9% NaCl	10 ML/HR
250-350	0.9% NaCl	10 ML/HR
200-249	0.9% NaCl + 2.5% DEXTROSE	7 ML/HR
150-199	0.9% NaCl + 2.5% DEXTROSE	5 ML/HR
100-149	0.9% NaCl + 5% DEXTROSE	5 ML/HR
<100	0.9% NaCl + 5% DEXTROSE	STOP INSULIN CRI

IV BAYTRIL (ENROFLOXACIN) DILUTION

DILUTE 1:4 to 1:10 (HOSPITAL DEPENDENT)

Remember that dilution ratios are added together for the total amount of parts.

EXAMPLE

1:4 = 5 PARTS
1:10 = 11 PARTS

EXAMPLE

BAYTRIL DOSAGE: 8.9 ML 1:4 DILUTION
8.9 ML = 1 PART OF 5 TOTAL PARTS
8.9 ML X 4 = 35.6 ML TOTAL VOLUME = 5 PARTS
       - 8.9 ML BAYTRIL = 1 PART
        26.7 ML DILUENT = 4 PARTS

INSTRUCTIONS:

1. Then place on syringe pump with separate line, stopping IVF's since Baytril is incompatible with most fluids.
2. Give TOTAL over 30 minutes.
3. 35.6 ML over 30 minutes is 71.2 ML/HR.

IV DOXYCYCLINE RECONSTITUTION & DILUTION

DILUTE 1:10

ORDER: 5 MG/KG IV BID
WEIGHT: 40.6 KG
RATE: X
TIME: 1 HR
CONC.: 100 MG/ML, RECONSTITUTE WITH 10ML 0.9% NaCl = 10 MG/ML THEN DILUTE 1:10 TO 1 MG/ML

DOXYCYCLINE DOSAGE:
5 MG/KG X 40.6 KG = 203 MG
203 MG / 10 MG/ML = 20.3 ML DOXY
20.3 ML X 11 = 223.3 ML TOTAL VOLUME = 11 PARTS
$\qquad$ -20.3 ML DOXY = 1 PART
$\qquad$ 203 ML DILUENT = 10 PARTS

DILUENT CHOICE: 250 ML IVF BAG OF 0.9% NaCl

RATE: 223.3 ML X 1 HR = 223.3 ML/HR = 223 ML/HR

INSTRUCTIONS:

1. Use 250 ML bag of 0.9% NaCl and remove 47 ML of saline first. (250 ML – 203 ML = 47 ML DILUENT).

2. Add 20.3 MLS 10 MG/ML Doxycycline to 203 ML DILUENT.

3. Ask your DVM if they would like to stop IVF therapy during infusion because it is preferable so as to not fluid overload the patient.

DIVIDING A DRUG INTO 2 60 ML SYRINGES

DRUG: DOXYCYCLINE
ORDER: 5 MG/KG IV BID
WEIGHT: 18 KG
RATE: X
TIME: 1 HR
CONC.: 100 MG/ML, RECONSTITUTE WITH 10 ML 0.9% NaCl = 10 MG/ML THEN DILUTE 1:10 TO 1 MG/ML

5 MG/KG X 18 KG = 90 MG
90 MG / 10 MG/ML = 9 ML DOXY
9ML DOXY x 11 = 99 ML TOTAL VOLUME
                    - 9 ML DOXY
                    90 ML DILUENT
99 ML / 2 SYRINGES = 49.5 ML/SYRINGE
9 ML DOXY / 2 SYRINGES = 4.5 ML DOXY/SYRINGE
90 ML DILUENT / 2 SYRINGES = 45 ML DILUENT/SYRINGE

RATE: 49.5 ML/SYRINGE X 2 = 99 ML/HR

This infusion is over 1 hour, so we would need to set each syringe to infuse over 30 minutes, so each 49.5 ML syringe would go on the syringe pump at 99 ML/HR.

N-ACETYLCYSTEINE - DILUTE

FOR ACETAMINOPHEN TOXICITY

ORDER: 140 MG/KG LOADING DOSE ONCE

      70 MG/KG DOSAGE Q6H X 7 TREATMENTS

WEIGHT: 30 KG

RATE: X

FLUIDS: Y

TIME: 20 MINS – GIVE SLOW IV

CONC: 20% = 200 MG/ML, DILUTE TO 5% = 50 MG/ML BY DILUTING 1:4 WITH 0.45% NaCl, STERILE H2O OR D5W AND USE A 0.22 MICRON FILTER AT PORT CLOSEST TO PATIENT

LOADING DOSE:

140 MG/~~KG~~ X 30 ~~KG~~ = 4200 MG

4200 ~~MG~~ / 200 ~~MG~~/ML = 21 ML NAC

LOADING DOSE DILUTION:

21 ML NAC 1:4 IN 0.45% NaCl, STERILE H2O OR D5W
REMEMBER 1:4 IS 5 TOTAL PARTS

21 ML X 5 = 105 ML TOTAL VOLUME – 5 PARTS

      <u>- 21 ML</u> NAC – 1 PART

      84 ML 0.45% NaCl, STERILE H2O OR D5W –

      4 PARTS = FLUIDS = Y

60 ~~MIN~~ / 20 ~~MIN~~ = 3 *THIS IS A UNIT OF TIME SO YOU WILL GET A RATE IN ML/HR WHEN CALCULATING

105 ML X 3 = 315 ML/HR = RATE = X

ADDITIONAL DOSES:

70 MG/KG X 30 KG = 2100 MG

2100 MG / 200 MG/ML = 10.5 ML NAC

10.5 ML X 5 = 52.5 ML TOTAL VOLUME - 5 PARTS

             - 10.5 ML NAC – 1 PART

                 42 ML 0.45% NaCl, STERILE H2O OR D5W

                     – 4 PARTS = FLUIDS = Y

60 ~~MIN~~ / 20 ~~MIN~~ = 3

52.5 ML X 3 = 157.5 ML/HR = RATE = X

NOTE: N-ACETYLCYSTEINE CONTAINS SODIUM AND TO PREVENT EXCESS SODIUM AND FLUID CREEP OVER THE COURSE OF HOSPITALIZATION IT IS RECOMMENDED NOT TO DILUTE WITH 0.9% NaCl BUT RATHER 0.45% NaCl, STERILE H2O or D5W.

IV DEXDOMITOR + IM ANTISEDAN CALCULATION

DEXDOMITOR 0.5 MG/ML DOSAGES ALWAYS EQUAL	ANTISEDAN 5 MG/ML ALWAYS IM UNLESS DIRECTED OTHERWISE
DOSAGE = 0.005 MG/KG	DOSAGE = 0.05 MG/KG
12 KG	12 KG
0.005 MG/KG X 12 KG = 0.06 MG	0.05 MG/KG X 12 KG = 0.6 MG
0.06 MG / 0.5 MG/ML = 0.12 ML DEXDOMITOR	0.6 MG / 5 MG/ML = 0.12 ML ANTISEDAN

DEXDOMITOR 500 MCG/ML DOSAGES ALWAYS EQUAL	ANTISEDAN 5000 MCG/ML ALWAYS IM UNLESS DIRECTED OTHERWISE
DOSAGE = 5 MCG/KG	DOSAGE = 50 MCG/KG
12 KG	12 KG
5 MCG/KG X 12 KG = 60 MCG	50 MCG/KG X 12 KG = 600 MCG
60 MCG / 500 MG/ML = 0.12 ML DEXDOMITOR	600 MCG / 5000 MCG/ML = 0.12 ML ANTISEDAN

DEXDOMITOR CRI (DILUTE - MCG/KG/HR)

ORDER: 2 MCG/KG/HR
WEIGHT: 28.8 KG
RATE: RUN AT 2 ML/HR
TIME: 10 HR
CONC.: 500 MCG/ML = 0.5 MG/ML

CALCULATE YOUR CRI:

2 MCG/~~KG~~/HR X 28.8 ~~KG~~ = 57.6 MCG/HR
57.6 MCG/~~HR~~ X 10 ~~HR~~ = 576 MCG
576 ~~MCG~~ / 500 ~~MCG~~/ML = 1.152 ML DEXDOMITOR

DILUTION:

2 ML/~~HR~~ X 10 ~~HR~~ = 20 ML TOTAL VOLUME
20 ML – 1.152 ML = 18.85 ML 0.9% NaCl

PROPOFOL CRI (STRAIGHT - MG/KG/MIN)

ORDER: 0.1 MG/KG/MIN
WEIGHT: 1.6 KG
RATE: X
TIME: 4 HR
CONC.: 10 MG/ML

CALCULATE YOUR CRI:

0.1 MG/~~KG~~/MIN X 1.6 ~~KG~~ = 0.16 MG/MIN
0.16 MG/~~MIN~~ X 60 ~~MIN~~/HR = 9.6 MG/HR
9.6 MG/~~HR~~ X 4 ~~HR~~ = 38.4 MG
38.4 ~~MG~~ / 10 ~~MG~~/ML = 3.84 ML TOTAL VOLUME

CALCULATE YOUR RATE:

3.84 ML / 4 HR = 0.96 ML/HR = RATE = X

CHAPTER 11:
20% MANNITOL

MANNITOL - 20% CONCENTRATION

DOSAGE: 0.5 G/KG – 1 G/KG = 500 MG/KG – 1000 MG/KG IV OR IO OVER 15 – 20 MINUTES Q6-8H PRN

CRI'S NOT RECOMMENDED

$\geq$15% MANNITOL IS A HYPEROSMOLAR AGENT

MONITORING: SERUM ELECTROLYTES (ESPECIALLY SODIUM)

OSMOLALITY (ESPECIALLY IF MULTIPLE DOSES OR CRI INITIATED)

BUN/SERUM CREATININE

URINE OUTPUT

CENTRAL VENOUS PRESSURE

LUNG AUSCULTATION

NEUROLOGICAL STATUS

ORDER: 0.5 G/KG = 500 MG/KG

WEIGHT: 12 KG

CONC: 20% = 200 MG/ML

500 MG/~~KG~~ X 12 ~~KG~~ = 6,000 MG

6,000 ~~MG~~ / 200 ~~MG~~/ML = 30 ML 20% MANNITOL

Instructions:

1. Use a filter needle with a 0.22 micron in-line filter when drawing up Mannitol.
2. Place a 0.22 micron in-line filter in the port closest to the patient and change the filter after every 50 MLS of Mannitol delivered.
3. Use a dedicated extension set, and if a Y-set is in place utilize the same port for repeat doses of Mannitol.
4. DO NOT give Mannitol that has crystallized.
5. DO NOT exceed 3 G/KG total dosage in 24 hours.
6. Elevate the patient's head 15 - 30 degrees to help decrease intracranial pressure.

CHAPTER 12: URINARY OUTPUT, SENSIBLE & INSENSIBLE LOSSES

CALCULATING URINARY OUTPUT WITH SENSIBLE AND INSENSIBLE LOSSES

CALCULATING IN'S

FLUID RATE X # OF HOURS = IN'S

CALCULATING OUT'S

SENSIBLE = HOW MANY MLS OF URINE

INSENSIBLE = 1/3 MAINTENANCE X # OF HOURS = MLS

TO CALCULATE 1/3 MAINTENANCE:

K9 = 60 ML/KG/DAY x 0.33

FELINE = 40 ML/KG/DAY x 0.33

CALCULATING UOP

TOTAL SENSIBLE OUT'S / WEIGHT (KGS) / # OF HOURS

EXAMPLE

28.8 KG DOG HAS A URINARY OUTPUT MEASURED AT 260 ML WITH A IVF RATE OF 150 ML/HR AND IT IS MEASURED Q4H.

150 ML/~~HR~~ X 4 ~~HR~~ = 600 ML

IN'S = 600 ML
OUT'S = SENSIBLE: 260 ML

1/3 MAINTENANCE CALCULATION:

60 ML/KG/DAY / 3 = 20 ML/KG/DAY
20 ML/~~KG~~/DAY X 28.8 ~~KG~~ = 576 ML/DAY
576 ML/~~DAY~~ / 24 HR/~~DAY~~ = 24 ML/HR
24 ML/~~HR~~ X 4 ~~HR~~ = 96 ML

INSENSIBLE: 96 ML

UOP = SENSIBLE OUT'S / WEIGHT (KG) / TIME = ML/KG/HR

UOP = 260 ML / 28.8 KG / 4 HR = 2.256 ML/KG/HR

CHAPTER 13:
HOW TO PLACE A MODIFIED ROBERT JONES BANDAGE

How to Place a Modified Robert Jones Bandage

Article by Brian Goleman, RVT of Brian's Bandages

Introduction: An original Robert Jones bandage was named for the World War I doctor who developed it. It was designed to aid soldiers wounded in battle. It is a very bulky bandage that offers compression and stabilization for wounds and/or broken limbs. In today's veterinary field, the original Robert Jones bandage is typically only found in the equine world. In small animal practices you will find a Modified Robert Jones, or MRJ. The MRJ is similar to the Robert Jones, except less cotton layer is applied, thus significantly decreasing the size of the bandage. The Modified Robert Jones bandage provides the same advantages as the Robert Jones bandage, yet it is more economical and tolerable for the patient.

Indications: Typically an MRJ will be used in the small animal field to aid with post-operative swelling, to stabilize a broken or luxated distal portion of a limb, or to protect a wound.

Contraindications: MRJ's should never be used on femur or humeral fractures as they cannot go high enough to stabilize the bone.

Supplies:

Stockinette
Cast padding
Cling wrap/Roll gauze
Vet wrap
Porous tape
Waterproof tape
Tongue depressor
+/- Wound dressing
+/- External coaptation

Step 1:
Shave the limb. When bandaging over hair, the bandage will be less likely to slip off the oily fur and our **porous tape stirrups** will stick better to the patient's skin rather than their fur.

Step 2:
Tape stirrups are the hero in keeping a bandage on. Place two pieces of tape on either side of the distal part of the limb and do not go above any joints that may be involved. To keep the stirrups from sticking to each other or getting tangled, attach the tape to a **tongue depressor**.

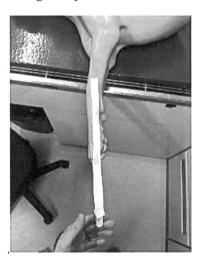

Step 3:
Begin wrapping your **cast padding** by starting a bit past the toes. This will give you good padding in the end. Ensure your wrap is loose enough to not cut off circulation but tight enough that the bandage does not slip off. The wrap should be even and consistent throughout the bandage. The result should look cylindrical and uniform.

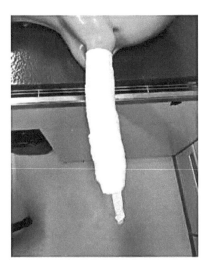

Step 4:
One or two layers of **cling wrap/roll gauze** should be applied with the same technique as **Step 3**. This step helps hold the cast padding in place. If an **external coaptation** is indicated, it would be applied at this step. Once the cling wrap is done, untape your stirrups and tape them up and attach them to your cling wrap.

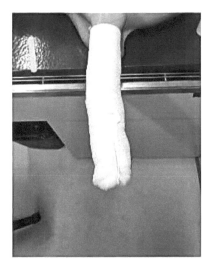

Step 5:
The top layer, the **vet wrap**, is applied. Just like in **Step 1**, begin

How to Place a Modified Robert Jones Bandage

Article by Brian Goleman, RVT of Brian's Bandages

begin wrapping the vet wrap a bit below the toes. Begin wrapping the vet wrap up with 50% overlap. Once you reach the top of the bandage, wrap back down with a 10% overlap. This layer protects the bandage from everyday dirt but also allows the bandage to breathe.

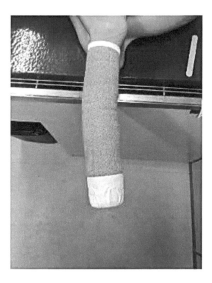

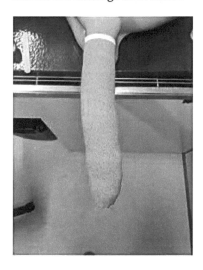

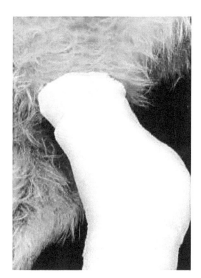

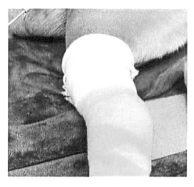

Step 6:
Most MRJ bandages will be open toed bandages so owners and the veterinary team can monitor for swelling. Use your **tongue depressor** to tuck in the excess bandage hanging below the toes and use waterproof tape to expose the toes. Make sure the toes do not stick out of the bandage. The goal is to have the patient walking on the bandage, not the toes. A closed-toe MRJ would be indicated if toe wounds or fractures were involved.

Photos Courtesy of:
Brian Goleman © 2023 and
Kristin Lake © 2022

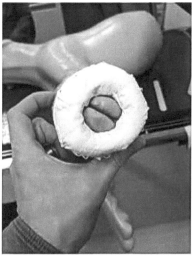

Pro Tip:
Use a **stockinette** at the top of your MRJ bandage. This would be slipped on as the first layer and would extend proximally above where the top of the bandage would terminate, and then would fold down over the **cling wrap/roll gauze** layer. **Stockinette** can really clean up the presentation of your bandage and it adds additional comfort for the patient.

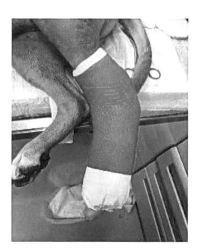

CHAPTER 14:
VENOMVET SNAKE BITE ENVENOMATION PROTOCOL

VENOMVET™
SNAKE BITE ENVENOMATION PROTOCOL
FOR CROTALIDS
BY KRISTIN LAKE, B.Sc. &
ASHLEY JOYCE, C.V.T.

KEEP IN REFRIGERATOR UNTIL READY FOR USE

DILUTION/ADMINISTRATION:

It is recommended to mix each vial of antivenin with 100ml – 150mls of a crystalloid fluid and administer IV slowly while taking into consideration the patient's weight and overall fluid load. Completed infusions can be reached at 30 minutes – 1 hour. VETGirl and the VenomVet Rep recommends 30 minute infusions unless contraindicated due to possibility for fluid overload, cardiac or renal impairment.

As with other equine derived antivenins, monitor the patient closely over the first 10 minutes for signs of hypersensitivity reactions. If one occurs then stop the infusion and re-assess the patient, when safe continue the transfusion at a lower rate.

ADVERSE REACTIONS:

As with any equine derived antivenin, adverse reactions may occur, including life threatening anaphylactic and anaphylactoid reactions. Medical veterinary care must be available during and after the administration of **VenomVet™**. Anaphylactic (Type 1 Hypersensitivity) and anaphylactoid reactions may be characterized by hypotension, respiratory distress, vomiting, diarrhea, angioedema, urticaria and wheals, pruritis and fever. Delayed hypersensitivity reactions can also occur requiring patient monitoring post-treatment.

Q: Can VenomVet™ be used to treat animals other than canines?

A: VenomVet™ is approved for use in treating canines only. No clinical trials were conducted using other animals. Used to treat dogs 6 months of age and older. There is no established evidence for treatment of cats.

Q: What are the storage conditions for VenomVet™?

A: Because VenomVet™ only requires refrigeration between 36 and 46 degrees Fahrenheit it is ready to use immediately and requires no mixing and waiting as with all other antivenin products on the market. So, REFRIGERATE. It does not need to come to room temperature. It is recommended that the product not be frozen.

Q: Can VenomVet™ only be administered with sterile saline?

A: The product insert recommends the administration of VenomVet™ with a crystalloid fluid.
Crystalloids

- Lactated Ringer's/Hartman's solution (lactate buffered solution)
- Acetate buffered solution
- Acetate and lactate buffered solution
- Acetate and gluconate buffered solution
- 0.45% NaCl (hypotonic solution)
- 0.9% NaCl (isotonic solution)
- 3% NaCl (hypertonic solution)
- 5% Dextrose in water
- 10% Dextrose in water

Q: How does a veterinarian determine whether to give VenomVet™ over 30 or 60 minutes?

A: The rate of infusion depends on the size of the animal. Faster infusion is the better choice but the veterinarian needs to avoid/control liquid overdose. Also the first milliliters should be administered slowly to check the appearance of secondary reactions.

Q: What technology does VenomVet™ use to combat the effects of Crotalid venin toxins?

A: VenomVet™ is obtained from the blood of healthy horses that have been immunized with Crotalid venoms. It is a polyvalent antivenin treatment that is produced under sterile and nonpyrogenic conditions using F(ab)2 Technology. Third party research provides that F(ab)2 is created by a pepsin digestion of purified IgG. It has a longer half-life and remains in the vascular compartment longer than F(ab) technology based products. Another significant difference is that it has two antigen binding sites per molecule and works by binding and neutralizing venom toxins. Once neutralized, it facilitates the redistribution of the neutralized toxins away from target tissues and they are then eliminated from the body.

From a safety standpoint the technology fully eliminates the Fc fragment. This significantly reduces hypersensitivity reactions during administration to envenomation victims.

TRIAGE & EMERGENCY STABILIZATION OF SNAKE BITE ENVENOMATIONS

TRIAGE

IF STABLE:

HAVE TEAM MATES GURNEY THE PET INSIDE AND PREVENT ANIMAL FROM MOBILIZING, TIME IS A FACTOR AND VENOM CAN REACH CENTRAL CIRCULATION FASTER IF THE ANIMAL IS MOBILE BEFORE TREATMENT IS INITIATED

TAKE COMPREHENSIVE HISTORY FROM OWNER INCLUDING DESCRIPTION OF SNAKE IF SEEN AND AREAS WHERE BITES MAY BE LOCATED

TIMEFRAME OF ENVENOMATION AND TIME ELAPSED SINCE ENVENOMATION IF ANY FIRST AID WAS ADMINISTERED AND WHAT KIND

NAMES AND DOSAGES OF ANY MEDICATIONS GIVEN AND ANY MEDICATIONS REGULARLY TAKEN AND FOR WHAT CONDITIONS

PREVIOUS PERTINENT MEDICAL HISTORY

SYMPTOMS DISPLAYED AND TIME OF ONSET AND LONGEVITY

FULL TPR WITH WEIGHT

PHYSICAL EXAMINATION BY DOCTOR

FULL BODY CHECK FOR BITE WOUNDS

IV CATHETER PLACEMENT - IDEALLY 2 PERIPHERAL IVC'S TO START ON 2 DIFFERENT NON-AFFECTED LIMBS - ONE DEDICATED TO VENOMVET, THE OTHER FOR A BLOOD DRAW OFF OF THE CATHETER FOR DIAGNOSTICS, IVF RESUSCITATION, AND POTENTIALLY FRESH FROZEN PLASMA. PLACE AN APPROPRIATE SIZE CATHETER TO THE PATIENT. - REMEMBER BITE WOUNDS MAY BE SMALL AND DIFFICULT TO VISUALIZE SO SHAVE AREAS THOROUGHLY AND EXAMINE BRIEFLY BUT THOROUGHLY BEFORE ASEPTIC TECHNIQUE FOR IVC PLACEMENT, TWO SETS OF EYES ARE BEST BUT IF YOU'RE 200% POSITIVE THERE ARE NO BITE WOUNDS WORK QUICKLY TO GET A CATHETER IN.

IF ONE LIMB IS AVAILABLE - PLACE A PERIPHERAL IVC IN IT AS SOON AS POSSIBLE AND BEGIN IV FLUID RESUSCITATION IN THAT LINE WHEN ORDERED BY THE DOCTOR. CONSIDER TRIPLE LUMEN CENTRAL LINE FOR SAMPLING, VENOMVET, IVF RESUSCITATION AND BLOOD PRODUCTS. (WORST CASE SCENARIO)

IF TWO LIMBS ARE AVAILABLE (EX. BITES ON MULTIPLE LIMBS) – PLACE 1-2 PERIPHERAL IVC'S FOR VENOMVET, IVF RESUSCITATION AND +/- BLOOD PRODUCTS.

IF THREE LIMBS ARE AVAILABLE - PLACE 1-2 PERIPHERAL IVC'S FOR VENOMVET, IVF RESUSCITATION AND +/- BLOOD PRODUCTS. +/- A PICC LINE FOR SAMPLING SO WE ARE NOT POKING THIS ANIMAL FOR BLOOD DRAWS AS IT MAY DEVELOP A COAGULOPATHY. (WORST CASE SCENARIO)

ASK DOCTOR FOR VERIFICATION OF LOCATIONS FOR IVC'S BEFORE PLACEMENT TO ENSURE NO AFFECTED LIMBS ARE BEING UTILIZED.

TRACE WITH BLACK MAGIC MARKER THE AFFECTED AREA AND MONITOR SITE REGULARLY AND UPDATE TRACING TO TRACK

SWELLING, LOCAL EDEMA, AND PROGRESSION OF LOCAL SYMPTOMS.

IF UNSTABLE:

ASK OWNER WHERE KNOWN BITES ARE LOCATED AS SOON AS POSSIBLE THEN BRING STRAIGHT BACK TO THE TREATMENT AREA

HAVE ANOTHER STAFF MEMBER DISCUSS HISTORICAL ITEMS WITH OWNER TAKING DETAILED NOTES AND ASKING THE QUESTIONS UNDER THE STABLE TRIAGE SECTION WHILE YOU AND THE REST OF THE TEAM BEGIN EMERGENCY STABILIZATION PROCEDURES

EMERGENCY STABILIZATION

ABC ASSESSMENT – IF AIRWAY COMPROMISED – ATTEMPT INTUBATION, IF UNABLE CONSIDER EMERGENCY TRACHEOSTOMY. IF BREATHING AND CIRCULATION COMPROMISED - START COMPRESSIONS AND INTUBATE AT THIS TIME WITH ETCO2 HOOKED UP TO MULTIPARAMETER MONITOR, PERFORM ONE ROUND OF 2 MINUTE COMPRESSIONS THEN ASSESS PATIENT FOR ROSC, IF ROSC IS ACHIEVED THEN BEGIN POST-ARREST CARE, IF ROSC IS NOT ACHIEVED, BEGIN ALS IMMEDIATELY AFTER ASSESSMENT.

ECG - LEADS ON WITH ULTRASOUND GEL - MONITOR FOR VPC'S, AIVR, V TACH, PVT, V-FIB AND ANY OTHER ABNORMALITIES.

BP - OSCILLOMETRIC BP CUFF ON MULTIPARAMETER MONITOR ON AND RUNNING SERIAL BP'S EVERY FEW MINUTES.

BRIEF PHYSICAL EXAM ON EXAM TABLE AND BRIEF CHECK FOR BITE WOUNDS BEFORE UTILIZING LIMBS FOR PERIPHERAL IVC

ACCESS - REMEMBER BITE WOUNDS MAY BE SMALL AND DIFFICULT TO VISUALIZE SO SHAVE AREAS THOROUGHLY AND EXAMINE BRIEFLY BUT THOROUGHLY BEFORE ASEPTIC TECHNIQUE FOR IVC PLACEMENT, TWO SETS OF EYES ARE BEST BUT IF YOU'RE 200% POSITIVE THERE ARE NO BITE WOUNDS WORK QUICKLY TO GET A CATHETER IN.

PLACE 1-2 IVC'S IN NON-AFFECTED LIMBS DEPENDING UPON DOCTOR'S ORDERS

BLOOD DRAW OFF OF CATHETER FOR CHEM/CBC/LYTES, PCV/TS, LACTATE, BG, AND TO CREATE A STAINED BLOOD SMEAR FOR IMMEDIATE ANALYSIS (LOOKING FOR RBC ECHINOCYTOSIS BUT CRENATION CAN HAPPEN TO SAMPLES THAT ARE ALLOWED TO SIT ON THE ROCKER IN AN EDTA TUBE AND "AGE" AND IS ALSO SEEN IN SAMPLES THAT HAVE BEEN UNDERFILLED IN THE EDTA TUBE, SO COLLECT THE PROPER AMOUNT AS WELL AND RUN RIGHT AWAY)

TFAST - EVALUATING FOR SIGNS OF HEMOTHORAX (BLOOD IN THE THORACIC CAVITY), AS CROTALID VENOM IS HEMOTOXIC, CYTOTOXIC, MYOTOXIC, AND LESS COMMONLY NEUROTOXIC. HYPOVOLEMIA (A SMALLER THAN NORMAL HEART CAN INDICATE DECREASED BLOOD VOLUME) AND RULING OUT ANY OTHER ABNORMALITIES. TXR MAY BE WARRANTED IF ABNORMALITIES FOUND ON TFAST.

IF HYPOVOLEMIC SHOCK IS SUSPECTED, INITIATE SHOCK BOLUS ALIQUOTS UNDER DOCTOR'S ORDERS WITH CRYSTALLOID FLUID.

PULSE OX - IF THE GODS ALLOW IT, BUT ABSOLUTELY TRY.

COMPLETE THE TPR WITH WEIGHT - WHEN STABLE OR ABLE. TO VISUALIZE THE PATIENT'S WEIGHT, THINK OF A LEAN, YOUNG 22LB BEAGLE AND THE SIZE THAT THIS WOULD BE. 22LB = 10KG HOW MANY BEAGLES WOULD IT TAKE TO BE THIS ANIMAL IN FRONT OF

YOU? LET'S SAY IT'S REALLY A 19KG K9, LOOKING AT HIM AND EYEBALLING IT, IT WOULD TAKE ABOUT 2 BEAGLES TO MAKE UP THIS PATIENT SO THAT MEANS 10KG PER BEAGLE = 20KG PATIENT. USE THIS AS A GUIDE TO ESTIMATE WEIGHT FOR UNSTABLE PATIENTS.

+/- TXR - WHEN STABLE OR ABLE - EVALUATING FOR SIGNS OF HEMOTHORAX (BLOOD IN THE THORACIC CAVITY) AND SEVERITY AS CROTALID VENOM IS HEMOTOXIC, CYTOTOXIC, MYOTOXIC, AND LESS COMMONLY NEUROTOXIC. ALSO EVALUATING FOR HYPOVOLEMIA (A SMALLER THAN NORMAL HEART CAN INDICATE DECREASED BLOOD VOLUME) AND RULING OUT ANY OTHER ABNORMALITIES.

BLOODWORK

1. BLOOD SMEAR - EVALUATE FOR SPHEROCYTES, ECHINOCYTES AND HEMOLYSIS - RUN IMMEDIATELY

Echinocytosis has been associated with rattlesnake envenomation in humans, cats, and dogs and can be used to aid in the diagnosis. Echinocytes are erythrocytes with uniform, regularly spaced membrane projections. Echinocyte formation is thought to be caused directly by the venom itself, is dose dependent, and is self limiting; morphologic changes resolve within 48 hours.

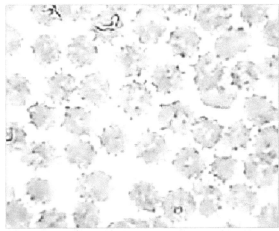

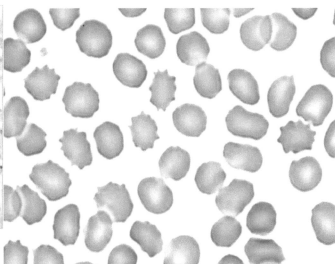

Figure 2. Echinocytosis on a blood smear following rattlesnake envenomation.

Echinocytosis

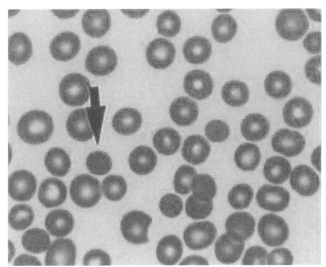

Spherocytosis of RBC

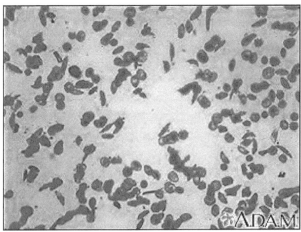

Hemolysis of RBCs – Also known as schistocytosis

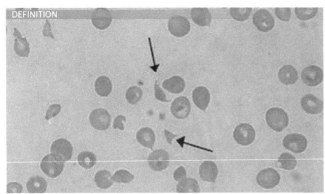

Hemolysis of RBCs – Also known as schistocytosis

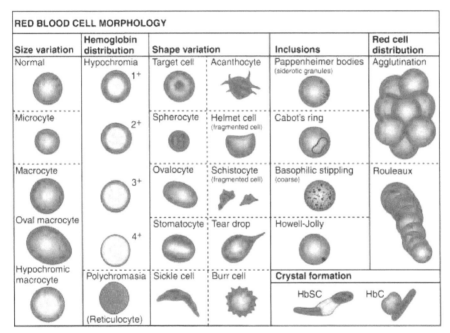

RBC Morphology

Spherocytosis and hemolysis noted after envenomation should be interpreted as signs of severe envenomation rather than as signs of immune-mediated hemolytic anemia.

Crenated RBCs are often found in blood smear's that have been dried for too long and "aging" of the blood in EDTA tube. Furthermore older RBCs that are nearing their half-life are more prone to this transformation into crenated configuration. More commonly, crenated RBCs are found in underfilled EDTA collection tubes and corrective actions such as making a new smear or re-collecting the sample must be performed.

2. COAGS (PT & aPTT) – COAGULOPATHY IS A CONCERN WITH CROTALID ENVENOMATIONS, PERFORM

3. PCV/TS – ALSO EVALUATE AND NOTATE SERUM COLOR FOR ICTERUS (YELLOW SERUM WHICH INDICATES INCREASED BILIRUBIN IN THE BLOOD INDICATING HEMOLYSIS/RBC DESTRUCTION). Continually monitor PCV/TS throughout course of hospitalization to ensure patient is not becoming anemic.

4. CBC – Laboratory abnormalities following envenomation include echinocytosis, thrombocytopenia, anemia or mild hemoconcentration, hypofibrinogenemia, elevated fibrin split products, leukocytosis, and prolonged clotting times. Serial blood testing should be conducted because the onset of coagulopathies can often be delayed.

5. CHEM17 – Chemistry profile changes that occur with rattlesnake envenomation include azotemia, hypoalbuminemia, hypoproteinemia, and elevated levels of creatinine kinase, alkaline phosphatase, alanine transaminase, g-glutamyl transferase, and aspartate transaminase.

6. LYTES – BASELINE NECESSARY SINCE WE UTILIZE ELECTROLYTE SOLUTIONS (0.9% SALINE OR D5W) FOR RECONSTITUTING DRUGS AND IVF'S CONTAIN ELECTROLYTES AS WELL. IF ADDITIVES ARE NECESSARY FOR CORRECTION WE NEED TO KNOW THAT TOO.

7. FULL URINALYSIS – RHABDOMYOLYSIS CAN OCCUR SECONDARY TO SNAKE BITE ENVENOMATIONS AND USUALLY CAUSES RED OR BROWN URINE FROM MYOGLOBINURIA AND/OR HEMOGLOBINURIA
Acute renal failure has been associated with snakebites in dogs.

The primary causes include the nephrotoxic effects of myoglobinuria and haemoglobinuria, DIC, toxic nephropathy and hypovolemic shock with renal ischemia. A FOLEY CATHETER MAY BE PRUDENT TO CONTINUALLY MONITOR FOR SIGNS OF RHABDOMYOLYSIS, HEMOLYSIS AND URINARY OUTPUT CALCULATION AND FOR RECUMBENT PATIENTS. (WORST CASE SCENARIO)

8. +/- LACTATE – IF HYPOVOLEMIC SHOCK OR PERFUSION DEFICITS ARE SUSPECTED OR DOCTOR ORDERS, THEN PERFORM

9. +/- BG ON GLUCOMETER – IF GLU DERANGED ON CHEM, IF PLANNING TO UTILIZE D5W OR DOCTOR ORDERS, THEN PERFORM

10. +/- BLOOD TYPE – IF BLOOD PRODUCTS ARE NEEDED

11. +/- MINOR CROSSMATCH – IF BLOOD PRODUCTS ARE NEEDED – BLOOD PRODUCTS UTILIZED ARE FRESH FROZEN PLASMA SO BE SURE TO UTILIZE THE MINOR CROSSMATCH (NOT THE MAJOR CROSSMATCH) WHICH TAKES DONOR PLASMA/SERUM AND FROM THE PIG TAILS OF THE FRESH FROZEN PLASMA BAG AND RECIPIENT WHOLE BLOOD TO ENSURE NO REACTION WILL HAPPEN FROM THE BLOOD TRANSFUSION.

12. +/- MAJOR CROSSMATCH – IF BLOOD PRODUCTS ARE NEEDED – BLOOD PRODUCTS UTILIZED FOR A PCV OR HCT THAT IS DROPPING OVER THE COURSE OF HOSPITALIZATION ARE PACKED RED BLOOD CELLS SO BE SURE TO UTILIZE THE MAJOR CROSSMATCH (NOT THE MINOR CROSSMATCH) WHICH TAKES DONOR ERYTHROCYTES FROM THE PIG TAILS OF THE PACKED RED BLOOD CELL BAG AND RECIPIENT SERUM TO ENSURE NO REACTION WILL HAPPEN FROM THE BLOOD TRANSFUSION.

IF WE ACHIEVE ROSC, HAVE 1-2 PATENT IVC'S, ECHINOCYTOSIS HAS BEEN CONFIRMED, OR IF PATIENT CAME IN STABLE, THEN START VENOMVET ON DOCTOR'S ORDERS AS SOON AS POSSIBLE OR WHEN IVF RESUSCITATION HAS TAKEN PLACE. IT TAKES ABOUT 30 MINUTES – 2 HOURS (DEPENDING ON SIZE OF PATIENT, SEVERITY OF ENVENOMATION, PROGRESSION OF SYMPTOMS, AND DOCTOR'S ORDERS) FOR EACH VIAL TO INFUSE. FACTOR THIS IN.

MANAGING HYPOTENSION DURING THE INFUSION OF VENOMVET:

"VENOMOUS ANIMALS USE VARIOUS ENVENOMATION STRATEGIES TO IMMOBILIZE, KILL AND COMMENCE THE DIGESTION OF PREY. BIOCHEMICAL MECHANISMS INVOLVED IN THE IMMOBILIZATION OF PREY ARE PARALYSIS AND/OR HYPOTENSION, WHICH LIMIT PREY FLIGHT AND RESISTANCE THROUGH DIRECT OR INDIRECT/SYNERGISTIC BIOCHEMICAL PROCESSES. IN ADDITION TO CIRCULATORY SHOCK AND RAPID PREY IMMOBILIZATION, HYPOTENSION MAY CONTRIBUTE TO THE DIFFUSION OF OTHER SNAKE VENOM COMPONENTS. PULMONARY VASCULAR OBSTRUCTION AND CORONARY ISCHEMIA CAUSED BY SNAKE VENOMS CAN FURTHER LEAD TO DECREASE IN BLOOD PRESSURE. PROTEINS AND PEPTIDES WITH DIRECT HYPOTENSIVE ACTIVITY EXERT THEIR ACTION BY BINDING TO SPECIFIC ENDOGENOUS MOLECULAR TARGETS (RECEPTORS, ENZYMES, CHANNELS)." SOURCE:
https://www.ncbi.nlm.nih.gov/pmc/articles/PMC6695636/#!po=15.0000

- GIVE 1/4 SHOCK DOSE ALIQUOTS UNTIL CLINICAL RESPONSE OR TOTAL SHOCK DOSE (40-60 ML/KG IN CATS; 60-90 ML/KG IN DOGS) IS REACHED IF NECESSARY. WATCH CLOSELY FOR FLUID OVERLOAD ESPECIALLY IF UTILIZING THE

HIGHER END OF THE DOSING RANGE.

- EPINEPHRINE OR NOREPINEPHRINE CRI IF REFRACTORY TO FLUID RESUSCITATION TITRATED UNTIL A MAP >65mmHg IS MET

- BEGIN MODIFIED GLASGOW COMA SCALE SCORING IF MENTATION BECOMES INAPPROPRIATE. HYPOPERFUSION TO THE BRAIN FROM SEVERE HYPOTENSION MAY CAUSE NEUROLOGICAL DEFICITS, BUT EASTERN DIAMONDBACK RATTLESNAKE ENVENOMATIONS MAY CAUSE NEUROLOGICAL SIGNS AS WELL. CNS SIGNS ARE GENERALLY NOT EXPECTED WITH COPPERHEAD AND COTTONMOUTH/WATER MOCCASIN ENVENOMATIONS.

- ASSESS FOR SIGNS OF CARDIOGENIC, HYPOVOLEMIC, ANAPHYLACTIC, AND/OR DISTRIBUTIVE/SEPTIC SHOCK, ESPECIALLY IN CASES OF A PROLONGED TIMEFRAME UNTIL MEDICAL CARE WAS ACCESSIBLE TO THE PATIENT

DVM TO ORDER ALL FLUID BOLUSES AND MEDICINAL INTERVENTIONS DURING INFUSION OF VENOMVET AFTER ASSESSING THE PATIENT. IF AT ANY TIME THE PATIENT IS UNSTABLE, STOP THE INFUSION, THEN WHEN DVM DIRECTS TO RESTART THE INFUSION, START AT A LOWER RATE. THIS WILL PROLONG THE INFUSION TIME, BUT STABILIZING THE PATIENT COMES FIRST.

MANAGING HYPERTENSION DURING THE INFUSION OF VENOMVET:

HYPERTENSION IS TYPICALLY ATTRIBUTED TO PAIN. OPIOIDS ARE THE DRUG CLASS OF CHOICE WITH NSAIDs TO BE AVOIDED. MORPHINE HOWEVER IS CONTRAINDICATED DUE TO THE POTENTIAL FOR HISTAMINE RELEASE.

Table 3

Snakebite severity score

Scoring should occur at presentation and at 6-hour intervals thereafter. Maximum possible score is 20. Risk of mortality increases with increasing scores

Snakebite Severity Score

System	Score	Signs
Respiratory	0	Normal
	1	Minimal: slight dyspnea
	2	Moderate: respiratory compromise, tachypnea, use of accessory muscles
	3	Severe: cyanosis, air hunger, extreme tachypnea, respiratory insufficiency or respiratory arrest from any cause
Cardiovascular	0	Normal
	1	Minimal: tachycardia, general weakness, benign dysrhythmia, hypertension
	2	Moderate: tachycardia, hyptension (tarsal pulse still palpable)
	3	Severe: extreme tachycardia, hypotension (nonpalpable tarsal pulse or systolic blood pressure < 80 mmHg), malignant dysrhythmia or cardiac arrest
Local Wound	0	Normal
	1	Minimal: pain, swelling, ecchymosis, erythema limited to bite site
	2	Moderate: pain, swelling, ecchymosis, erythema involves less than half of extremity and may be spreading slowly
	3	Severe: pain, swelling, ecchymosis, erythema involves most or all of one extremity and is spreading rapidly
	4	Very severe: pain, swelling, ecchymosis, erythema extends beyond affected extremity, or significant tissue necrosis
Gastrointestinal	0	Normal
	1	Minimal: abdominal pain, tenesmus
	2	Moderate: vomiting, diarrhea
	3	Severe: repetitive vomiting, diarrhea, or hematemesis
Hematological	0	Normal
	1	Minimal: coagulation parameters slightly abnormal, PT < 20 sec, PTT < 50 sec, platelets 100,000 to 150,000/mm3
	2	Moderate: coagulation parameters abnormal, PT 20-50 sec, PTT 50-75 sec, platelets 50,000 to 100,000/mm3
	3	Severe: coagulation parameters abnormal, PT 50-100 sec, PTT 75-100 sec, platelets 20,000 to 50,000/mm3
	4	Very severe: coagulation parameters markedly abnormal with bleeding present or the threat of spontaneous bleeding, including PT unmeasurable, PTT unmeasurable, platelets <20,000/mm3
Central Nervous System	0	Normal
	1	Minimal: apprehension
	2	Moderate: chills, weakness, faintness, ataxia
	3	Severe: lethargy, seizures, coma

Modified from Peterson ME. Snake bite: Pit vipers. Clin Techn Small Anim Pract 2006;21:177–8; with permission.

VenomVet Example:

20kg Canine
Order: 1 vial over 30 minutes
Fluids: 10ml VenomVet : 90ml crystalloid fluid = 100ml TOTAL

Time	Rate	VTBI	Math
Start-10 min mark	150ml/hr	25ml	0.125ml/kg/min = 2.5ml/min = 25ml infused over 10 minutes
10 min-20 min mark	150ml/hr	25ml	0.125ml/kg/min = 2.5ml/min = 25ml infused over 10 minutes
If NO reaction: 20 min-30 min mark	300ml/hr	50ml	0.25ml/kg/min = 5ml/min = 50ml infused over 10 minutes

The ML/KG/MIN may change per patient, thus the rate and VTBI will change as well. Start at a low rate, 0.125 - 0.25 ML/KG/MIN is a good jumping off point. Increase the rate every 10 minutes to get remainder in within 30 minutes. Check to ensure that you are within the daily fluid guidelines for that patient with your infusion.

60 ml/kg/day = 1xM *(Dehydration deficit not accounted for)*
60 ml/kg/day x 20 kg = 1200 ml/day
1200 ml/day / 24 hr/day = 50 ml/hr

1200 ml/day – 100 ml VenomVet dilution = 1100 ml/day so adjust fluid rate post-infusion: 1100 ml/day / 24 hr/day = 45.8 ml/hr

VenomVet Example:

20kg Canine
Order: 1 vial over 1 hour
Fluids: 10ml VenomVet : 90ml crystalloid fluid = 100ml TOTAL

Time	Rate	VTBI	Math
Start-10 min mark CHECK VITALS EVERY 5 MINUTES FOR A REACTION	75ml/hr	12.5ml	Start low and slow at 0.0625ml/kg/min x 20 kg = 1.25ml/min 1.25ml/min x 10 min = 12.5ml over 10 min = 75ml/hr
10 min-20 min mark CHECK VITALS EVERY 5 MINUTES FOR A REACTION	75ml/hr	12.5ml	0.0625ml/kg/min x 20 kg= 1.25ml/min 1.25ml/min x 10 min = 12.5ml over 10 min = 75ml/hr
If NO reaction: 20 min-30 min mark	90ml/hr	15ml	0.075ml/kg/min x 20 kg= 1.5ml/min 1.5ml/min x 10 min = 15ml over 10 min = 90ml/hr
30 min-40 min mark	120ml/hr	20ml	0.1ml/kg/min x 20 kg= 2 ml/min 2ml/min x 10 min = 20 ml over 10 min = 120ml/hr
40 min-50 min mark	120ml/hr	20ml	0.1ml/kg/min x 20 kg= 2 ml/min 2ml/min x 10 min = 20 ml over 10 min = 120ml/hr

50 min-60 min mark	120ml/hr	20ml	0.1ml/kg/min x 20 kg= 2 ml/min 2ml/min x 10 min = 20 ml over 10 min =120ml/hr

The ML/KG/MIN may change per patient, thus the rate and VTBI will change as well. Start at a low rate, 0.0625 - 0.25 ML/KG/MIN is a good jumping off point. Increase the rate every 10 minutes to get remainder in within 1 hour. Check to ensure that you are within the daily fluid guidelines for that patient with your infusion.

60 ml/kg/day = 1xM *(Dehydration deficit not accounted for)*
60 ml/kg/day x 20 kg = 1200 ml/day
1200 ml/day / 24 hr/day = 50 ml/hr

1200 ml/day – 100 ml VenomVet dilution = 1100 ml/day so adjust fluid rate post-infusion: 1100 ml/day / 24 hr/day = 45.8 ml/hr

It is the doctor's discretion regarding the rate of the infusion over 30 minutes - 2 hours. Have someone else double-check your math before beginning the infusion.

ADMINISTRATION TECHNIQUES:

2 Methods of Administration of 1 vial over 30 minutes - 2 hours:

1 100ML BAG OF CRYSTALLOID FLUID

USE A 12ML SYRINGE AND 18GA NEEDLE TO REMOVE 10ML FROM 100ML BAG CRYSTALLOID FLUID. USE A SECOND 12ML SYRINGE AND 18GA NEEDLE TO WITHDRAW 10ML VENOMVET INTO SYRINGE AND ADD 10ML VENOMVET TO 90ML (REMAINDER) BAG FOR 100ML TOTAL. SLOWLY FLUSH THE LENGTH OF THE LINE WITH 0.9% NaCl WHEN FINISHED WITH INFUSION.

OR

1 1L BAG OF CRYSTALLOID FLUID AND 1 BURETROL (AUTHOR'S FAVORITE METHOD)

IF 100ML BAGS ARE **NOT** AVAILABLE, USE A BURETROL WITH 1L OF CRYSTALLOID FLUID AND FILL BURETROL TO 90MLS AND ADD 10ML VENOMVET IN BURETROL. SLOWLY FLUSH THE LENGTH OF THE LINE WITH 0.9% NaCl WHEN FINISHED WITH INFUSION.

Consult doctor IMMEDIATELY for signs of hypersensitivity reactions/anaphylaxis, or if there is a progression of symptoms. Infusion may be slowed or stopped, emergency drugs may be utilized or a second vial may be instituted.

VENOMVET FOR CATS PROTOCOL BY KRISTIN LAKE, B.Sc. AND ASHLEY JOYCE, C.V.T.

VENOMVET WAS DESIGNED FOR CANINE USE ONLY WITH TESTING ONLY PERFORMED IN DOGS. IT IS ONLY VIA ANECDOTAL EVIDENCE AT THIS TIME FOR ITS USE IN CATS. OWNERS SHOULD BE MADE AWARE OF THIS AND ALLOWED TO DECIDE IF THEY WOULD LIKE VENOMVET TO BE GIVEN TO THEIR CAT.

ANECDOTALLY, I HAVE GIVEN THIS OVER ONE HOUR TO A FELINE (NOT 30 MINUTES DUE TO CONCERN FOR FLUID OVERLOAD AT THOSE RATES) WITH A COPPERHEAD SNAKE BITE ON THE CARPUS OF THE RIGHT FORELIMB WITH TWO CLEAR PUNCTURE WOUNDS THAT INDICATED A WIDTH THAT IS COMPARABLE TO AN ADULT COPPERHEAD, NOT A JUVENILE. PRE-INFUSION HIS BLOOD SMEAR SHOWED ECHINOCYTOSIS AND SCHISTOCYTOSIS. DURING THE INFUSION HE DEVELOPED PETECHIATION OF THE MUCOUS MEMBRANES AND SWELLING PERSISTED IN HIS LIMB THREE-FOURTH'S OF THE WAY THROUGH THE INFUSION. POST-INFUSION HE SHOWED NO EDEMA IN HIS LIMB OR INCREASED SWELLING, AND PETECHIATION WAS STATIC. POST-INFUSION BLOOD SMEAR SHOWED DRAMATIC DECREASE IN ECHINOCYTOSIS AND NO SCHISTOCYTOSIS. COAGS WERE NORMAL PRE- AND POST-INFUSION. HE DID HAVE A MILD HYPERSENSITIVITY REACTION MID-INFUSION AND WAS GIVEN 2MG/KG OF DIPHENHYDRAMINE IM. I STAYED AT THE 80ML/HR RATE FOR AN ADDITIONAL CYCLE UNTIL HIS TEMPERATURE WENT BACK DOWN AFTER SPIKING DURING MY Q5M VITALS CHECKS. THIS INCREASED HIS OVERALL INFUSION TIME, BUT WE HAD POSITIVE RESULTS. FOR PAIN, HE WAS GIVEN BUPRENORPHINE IV, GABAPENTIN PO, AND METHADONE IV PRE- AND

MID-INFUSION AND CONTINUED METHADONE IV Q4H AND GABAPENTIN PO Q8H POST-INFUSION. SNAKE BITE SEVERITY SCORE WAS 3 OUT OF 20 MID-INFUSION AND THIS INDICATED A VERY GOOD PROGNOSIS FOR THIS PATIENT.

ORDER: 10ML VENOMVET : 90ML 0.9% NaCl IN BURETROL
WEIGHT: 5.26 KG CAT
TIME: 1 HOUR

FOR THIS PATIENT, I STARTED LOW AND SLOW WITH 0.125 ML/KG/MIN AS A JUMPING OFF POINT, THEN DOUBLED IT TO 0.25 ML/KG/MIN THEN DOUBLED THAT TO 0.5 ML/KG/MIN:

TIME	RATE	VTBI
0-10 MIN	~40 ML/HR	6.6 ML = ~7 ML 0.125 ML/KG/MIN = 0.66 ML/MIN
10-20 MIN	~80ML/HR	13.15 ML = ~13 ML 0.25 ML/KG/MIN = 1.315 ML/MIN
20-30 MIN	~80 ML/HR	13.15 ML = ~13 ML 0.25 ML/KG/MIN = 1.315 ML/MIN
30-40 MIN	~80 ML/HR	13.15 ML = ~13 ML 0.25 ML/KG/MIN = 1.315 ML/MIN
40-50 MIN	~160 ML/HR - MAX RATE	26.3 ML = ~27 ML 0.5 ML/KG/MIN = 2.63 ML/MIN
50-60 MIN	~160 ML/HR - MAX RATE	26.3 ML = ~27 ML 0.5 ML/KG/MIN = 2.63 ML/MIN

TOTAL VOLUME INFUSED: 98.65 ML = 100.00 ML OVER ~1 HOUR

*IF HYPERSENSITIVITY REACTION OCCURS, STAY AT CURRENT RATE, ADMINISTER DIPHENHYDRAMINE IM AND/OR EPINEPHRINE IV AT DVM'S DISCRETION, MONITOR VITALS, AND WHEN VITALS ARE STABLE, DECIDE WHETHER TO INCREASE RATE DURING THE NEXT CYCLE OR TO EXTEND THE OVERALL INFUSION TIME AT THE CURRENT RATE.

FOR A MORE CONSERVATIVE APPROACH, START FELINE PATIENTS AT 0.1 ML/KG/MIN (~0.5 ML/MIN) AND EXTEND THE INFUSION TO TWO HOURS. THIS IS FOR FELINE PATIENTS WITHOUT CRITICAL NEED, WITH RENAL/CARDIAC IMPAIRMENT, PATIENTS HAVING OR ARE A CONCERN FOR HYPERSENSITIVITY REACTIONS, OR FOR PATIENTS THAT ARE A CONCERN FOR FLUID OVERLOAD.

ORDER: 10ML VENOMVET : 90ML 0.9% NaCl IN BURETROL
WEIGHT: 5.26 KG CAT
TIME: 2 HOURS

DOSAGE (ML/MIN)	VTBI (ML)	RATE (ML/HR)
0.1 ML/MIN	1	10
0.5 ML/MIN	5	30
0.75 ML/MIN	7.5	45
1 ML/MIN	10	60
1.25 ML/MIN	12.5	75
1.5 ML/MIN	15	90
1.75 ML/MIN	17.5	105
2 ML/MIN	20	120
2.25 ML/MIN	22.5	135
2.5 ML/MIN	25	150
3 ML/MIN	30	180
3.5 ML/MIN	35	210
4 ML/MIN	40	240
4.5 ML/MIN	45	270
5 ML/MIN	50	300

TIME	RATE	VTBI
0-10 MIN	30 ML/HR	0.5ML/MIN = 5ML
10-20 MIN	30 ML/HR	0.5ML/MIN = 5ML
20-30 MIN	45 ML/HR	0.75ML/MIN = 7.5 ML
30-40 MIN	45 ML/HR	0.75ML/MIN = 7.5 ML
40-50 MIN	45 ML/HR	0.75ML/MIN = 7.5 ML
50-60 MIN	45 ML/HR	0.75ML/MIN = 7.5 ML
60-70 MIN	60 ML/HR	1ML/MIN = 10 ML
70-80 MIN	60 ML/HR	1ML/MIN = 10 ML
80-90 MIN	60 ML/HR	1ML/MIN = 10 ML
90-100 MIN	60 ML/HR	1ML/MIN = 10 ML
100-110 MIN	60 ML/HR	1ML/MIN = 10 ML
110-120 MIN	60 ML/HR	1ML/MIN = 10 ML

TOTAL VOLUME INFUSED: 100.00 ML OVER 2 HOURS

Go to http://www.thevettechsguidetoecc.com for calculated Antivenin Rate Sheets over 30 minutes, 1 hour and 2 hours!

Emergency Drugs
Diphenhydramine 2mg/kg IM = _____ mL
Epinephrine 0.01mg/kg IV/IM = _____ mL
Epinephrine CRI 0.05 mcg/kg/min IV = _____ mL/hr

Antivenin Infusion Monitoring Form

Patient Name: _____

Start Date/Time: _____ End Date/Time: _____

Presentation Vitals: HR: _____ RR/RE: _____ MM/CRT: _____ Temp: _____ Weight: _____

BP: _____ PT/aPTT: _____ Blood Smear: _____

Time	Rate (mL/hr)	VTBI	HR	RR/RE	MM/CRT	Temp	BP	Snake Bite Severity Score	Notes
Start-10 minutes *CHECK EVERY 5 MINUTES FOR REACTION*	5m _____ 10m								
10-20 minutes *CHECK EVERY 5 MINUTES FOR REACTION*	15m _____ 20m								
20-30 minutes *CHECK EVERY 10 MINUTES FOR REACTION*									
30-40 minutes *CHECK EVERY 10 MINUTES FOR REACTION*									
40-50 minutes *CHECK EVERY 10 MINUTES FOR REACTION*									
50-60 minutes *CHECK EVERY 10 MINUTES FOR REACTION*									

Post-Infusion Vitals: HR: _____ RR/RE : _____ MM/CRT: _____ Temp: _____ Weight: _____

BP: _____ PT/aPTT: _____ Blood Smear: _____

Antivenin Reaction? Y   N Describe: _____   Emergency Drugs Given? Y   N

Notes: _____

_____

EPINEPHRINE CRI (DILUTE - MCG/KG/MIN)

FOR TREATMENT OF ANAPHYLAXIS

ORDER: 0.05 MCG/KG/MIN TO 0.4 MCG/KG/MIN
WEIGHT: 20 KG
RATE: RUN FROM 1 ML/HR AT 0.05 MCG/KG/MIN TO 8 ML/HR AT 0.4 MCG/KG/MIN
FLUID: Y
TIME: 1 HOUR WITH DOSE TITRATED UNTIL CLINICAL RESPONSE IS ACHIEVED
CONC.: 1 MG/ML

TITRATION EVERY 15 MINUTES FOR 1 HOUR:

60 MIN / 4 = 15 MIN

DIVIDE BY 4 BECAUSE WE WILL TITRATE UP AS FOLLOWS AND THERE ARE 4 TITRATION STEPS UNTIL MAXIMUM DOSAGE IS ACHIEVED:

0.05 MCG/KG/MIN   DOUBLE
0.1 MCG/KG/MIN   DOUBLE
0.2 MCG/KG/MIN   DOUBLE
0.4 MCG/KG/MIN

0.05 MCG/~~KG~~/MIN x 20 ~~KG~~ = 1 MCG/MIN
1 MCG/~~MIN~~ x 15 ~~MIN~~ = 15 MCG
15 ~~MCG~~/HR / 1000 ~~MCG~~/MG = 0.015 MG/HR
0.015 MG/~~HR~~ X 1 ~~HR~~ = 0.015 MG
0.015 ~~MG~~ / 1 ~~MG~~/ML = 0.015 ML EPINEPHRINE
0.015 ML X 1 HR = 0.015 ML/HR

0.015 ML + 0.03 ML + 0.06 ML +0.12 ML = 0.225 ML EPINEPHRINE
1 ML/HR + 2 ML/HR + 4 ML/HR + 8 ML/HR = 15 ML/HR T.V.
15 ML/HR - 0.225 ML = 14.775 ML/HR 0.9% NACL

SINCE THIS IS OVER 1 HOUR 15 ML IS OUR TOTAL VOLUME, 14.775 ML IS OUR DILUENT VOLUME, AND 0.225 ML IS OUR TOTAL EPINEPHRINE VOLUME.

TITRATION TABLE

TIME	DILUTED RATE	EPI RATE AT MCG/KG/MIN	EPINEPHRINE VOLUME
0-15 MINS	1 ML/HR	0.05 MCG/KG/MIN	0.015 ML
15-30 MINS	2 ML/HR	0.1 MCG/KG/MIN	0.03 ML
30-45 MINS	4 ML/HR	0.2 MCG/KG/MIN	0.06 ML
45-60 MINS	8 ML/HR	0.4 MCG/KG/MIN	0.12 ML

NOREPINEPHRINE CRI (DILUTE – MCG/KG/MIN)

FOR TREATMENT OF PERSISTENT HYPOTENSION AFTER ADEQUATE FLUID VOLUME REPLACEMENT

DOSAGE RANGE: 0.05-0.1 MCG/KG/MIN TITRATED UNTIL A MAP OF >65mmHg IS REACHED, MAX CRI RATE OF 1-2 MCG/KG/MIN (PLUMB'S)

ORDER: 0.05 MCG/KG/MIN TO START AND TITRATE UP TO 0.1 MCG/KG/MIN

WEIGHT: 20 KG

RATE: RUN @ 5 ML/HR FOR 0.05 MCG/KG/MIN - 10 ML/HR FOR 0.1 MCG/KG/MIN *PLAN TO TITRATE UP TO THE 10 ML/HR DOSE AS ORDERED BUT STAY AT THE RATE THAT ACHIEVES CLINICAL RESPONSE*

FLUIDS: Y

TIME: 1 HOUR WITH DOSE TITRATED UNTIL CLINICAL RESPONSE IS ACHIEVED

CONC.: 1 MG/ML

TITRATION EVERY 30 MINUTES FOR 1 HOUR:

0.05 MCG/~~KG~~/MIN X 20 ~~KG~~ = 1 MCG/MIN

1 MCG/~~MIN~~ X 30 ~~MIN~~ = 30 MCG

30 ~~MCG~~ / 1000 ~~MCG~~/MG = 0.03 MG

0.03 ~~MG~~ / 1 ~~MG~~/ML = 0.03 ML NOREPI FOR 30 MINS @ 0.05 MCG/KG/MIN

0.1 MCG/~~KG~~/MIN X 20 ~~KG~~ = 2 MCG/MIN

2 MCG/~~MIN~~ X 30 ~~MIN~~ = 60 MCG

60 ~~MCG~~ / 1000 ~~MCG~~/ML = 0.06 MG

0.06 ~~MG~~ / 1 ~~MG~~/ML = 0.06 ML NOREPI FOR 30 MINS @ 0.1 MCG/KG/MIN

5 ML + 10 ML = 15 ML T.V.

0.03 ML + 0.06 ML = 0.09 ML NOREPI

15 ML - 0.09 ML NOREPI = 14.91 ML 0.9% NACL

TITRATION TABLE

TIME	DILUTED RATE	NOREPI RATE AT MCG/KG/MIN	NOREPI VOLUME
START-30 MINS	5 ML/HR	0.05 MCG/KG/MIN	0.03 ML
30 MINS-60 MINS	10 ML/HR	0.1 MCG/KG/MIN	0.06 ML

INTERPRETING CANINE BLOOD TYPING KIT RESULTS

The Alvedia Canine DEA 1.1 Blood Typing Kits ALSO tests for DEA 1.2+ – It does not alert you to this on the kit, please follow these guidelines for interpretation

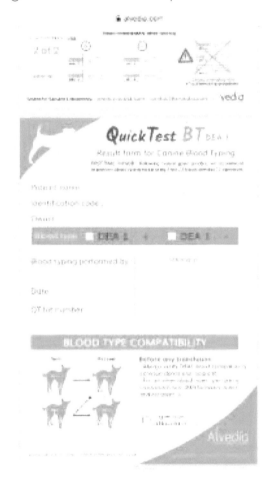

CANINE BLOOD TYPING
PROCEDURE

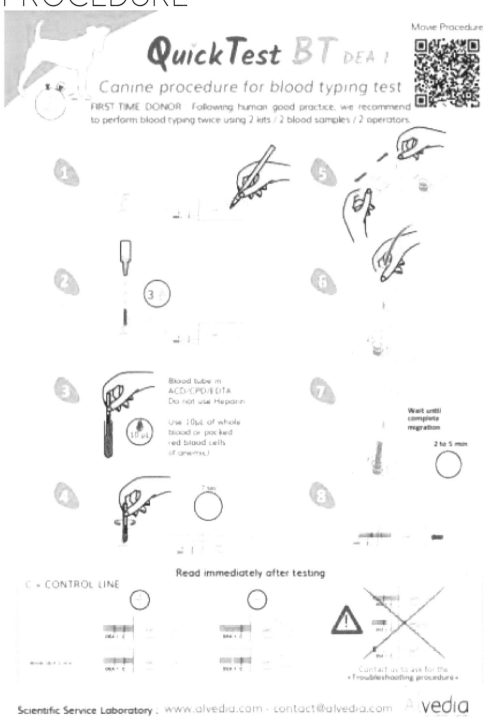

QuickTest BT DEA 1

Canine procedure for blood typing test

FIRST TIME DONOR Following human good practice, we recommend to perform blood typing twice using 2 kits / 2 blood samples / 2 operators.

Blood tube in ACD/CPD/EDTA
Do not use Heparin

Use 10µL of whole blood or packed red blood cells (if anemic)

Wait until complete migration

2 to 5 min

Read immediately after testing

C = CONTROL LINE

Contact us to ask for the « Troubleshooting procedure »

Scientific Service Laboratory : www.alvedia.com - contact@alvedia.com Alvedia

INTERPRETATION OF BLOOD TYPING RESULTS

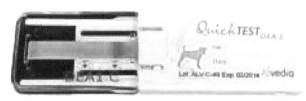

DEA 1.1 -

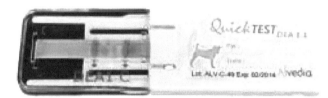

DEA 1.1 +

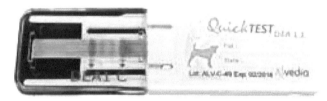

DEA 1.1 +

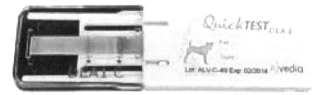

DEA 1.2 +

A strong or a weak positive indicates TWO different blood type results Strong Positive = DEA 1.1+
Weak Positive = DEA 1.2+ (DO NOT INFUSE WITH 1.1+ BLOOD PRODUCTS OR A REACTION CAN OCCUR)

AUTO-AGGLUTINATION CAN BE DETECTED BY THE CAPILLARY STRIP ON THE CANINE BLOOD TYPING TEST

RELIABLE IN CASE OF AUTO-AGGLUTINATION

Thanks to our specific membrane technology, the agglutinated red blood cells (RBCs) will be retained at the bottom of the membrane whereas non agglutinated RBCs will continue to migrate to the top of the membrane.

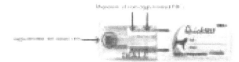

LOW PCV'S SHOULD GIVE ACCURATE RESULTS

RELIABLE IN CASE OF LOW PCV [ANEMIA]

Thanks to the sensivity of our specific monoclonal antibodies, even with a low pcv a reliable blood type can be obtained.

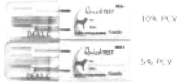

10% PCV

5% PCV

THESE WILL READ AS WEAK POSITIVES IF YOUR PATIENT HAS POSITIVE BLOOD. PERFORM A SLIDE AGGLUTINATION WITH DONOR AND RECIPIENT BLOOD PRODUCTS TO CONFIRM WHETHER A REACTION IS LIKELY TO HAPPEN.

MAJOR CROSSMATCH TESTING

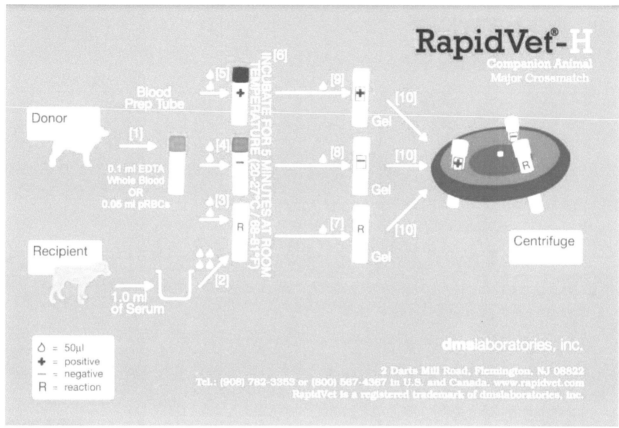

FIGURE 1.
RAPIDVET-H CROSSMATCH KIT

Interpreting and Reporting Results

Use the Crossmatch Photo Identifier provided to interpret results in Clear Top Negative (-) and Positive (+) Control Gel Tubes.

NEGATIVE CONTROL: Clear Top Negative (-) Control Gel Tube (green label) should demonstrate a collection of red blood cells at the **bottom** of the gel column.

POSITIVE CONTROL: Clear Top Positive (+) Control Gel Tube (red label) should demonstrate an agglutination of red blood cells at the top of the gel column or a dispersion of red cells mid matrix and above.

IMPORTANT: If controls do not react as stated above DO NOT proceed with the interpretation of test.

Crossmatch Photo Identifier

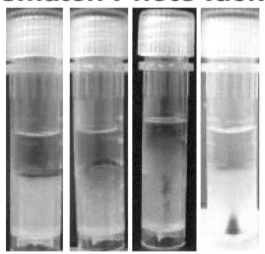

POSITIVE (Incompatible donor/recipient)

A positive test is considered any tube demonstrating red blood cells at or near the top of the gel column after centrifugation. In weak agglutinations, the cells may end up at the bottom of the tube in a conical or bell-shaped configuration. In this instance, the peak of the reaction will extend more than halfway up the gel column. **DO NOT TRANSFUSE USING THIS DONOR.**

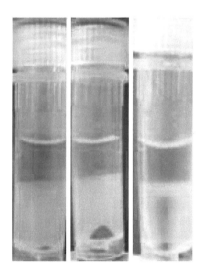

NEGATIVE (Compatible donor/recipient)

A negative test is considered any tube where the vast majority of red blood cells are at or near the bottom of the gel column after centrifugation and no firm line of agglutinated cells remains at the top of the gel. **IT IS UNLIKELY THAT A SIGNIFICANT REACTION WILL RESULT FROM A TRANSFUSION USING THIS DONOR.**

Rev. 12/2017

dmslaboratories, inc.
2 Darts Mill Road, Flemington, NJ 08822
Tel.: (908) 782-3353 or (800) 567-4367 in U.S. and Canada, Fax: (908) 782-0832
RapidVet is a registered trademark of **dms**laboratories, inc.

SALINE SLIDE AGGLUTINATION TEST

1 DROP OF WHOLE BLOOD
3-4 DROPS OF SALINE

.INSTRUCTIONS:

1. DROP BOTH WHOLE BLOOD AND SALINE ONTO A SLIDE.

2. ROCK BACK AND FORTH MIXING TOGETHER THOROUGHLY.

3. OBSERVE MACROSCOPICALLY FOR EVIDENCE OF AGGLUTINATION.

4. ANALYZE UNDER MICROSCOPE FOR ROULEAUX (COIN STACKING
APPEARANCE) VERSUS AGGLUTINATION (CLUMPING LIKE
BUNCHES OF GRAPES).

WHEN RED BLOOD CELL AGGLUTINATES ARE PRESENT IN A
SAMPLE THIS INDICATES A HEMOLYTIC ANEMIA.

MINOR CROSSMATCH SLIDE AGGLUTINATION TEST

2 DROPS DONOR PLASMA (FRESH FROZEN PLASMA - FROM PIG TAIL)
1 DROP RECIPIENT WHOLE BLOOD (EDTA TUBE)

INSTRUCTIONS:

1. DROP 2 DROPS DONOR PLASMA AND 1 DROP RECIPIENT WHOLE BLOOD ONTO A SLIDE.
2. ROCK BACK AND FORTH MIXING TOGETHER THOROUGHLY.
3. OBSERVE SLIDE MACROSCOPICALLY FOR EVIDENCE OF AGGLUTINATION.
4. ANALYZE UNDER MICROSCOPE FOR ROULEAUX (COIN STACKING APPEARANCE) VERSUS AGGLUTINATION (CLUMPING LIKE BUNCHES OF GRAPES).

MAJOR CROSSMATCH SLIDE AGGLUTINATION TEST

2 DROPS RECIPIENT PLASMA (SPUN DOWN SAMPLE
FROM SERUM SEPARATOR TUBE)
1 DROP DONOR BLOOD (pRBC's, FRESH WHOLE BLOOD –
FROM PIG TAIL)

INSTRUCTIONS:

1. DROP 2 DROPS RECIPIENT PLASMA AND 1 DROP DONOR BLOOD
ONTO A SLIDE.
2. ROCK BACK AND FORTH MIXING TOGETHER THOROUGHLY.
3. OBSERVE SLIDE MACROSCOPICALLY FOR
EVIDENCE OF AGGLUTINATION.
4. ANALYZE UNDER MICROSCOPE FOR ROULEAUX (COIN
STACKING APPEARANCE) VERSUS AGGLUTINATION (CLUMPING
LIKE BUNCHES OF GRAPES).

IF AGGLUTINATION IS NOTED ON MAJOR CROSSMATCH, DO
NOT PROCEED WITH TRANSFUSION. ANOTHER DONOR SHOULD
BE SELECTED. IF AGGLUTINATION IS NOTED ON MINOR
CROSSMATCH, PROCEED WITH CAUTION. IF POSSIBLE
ANOTHER DONOR SHOULD BE SELECTED.

CALCULATING BLOOD TRANSFUSION VOLUME FROM DONOR TO RECIPIENT

GIVEN:

DONOR WEIGHT: 27.7 KG

RECIPIENT WEIGHT: 30.3 KG

DESIRED PCV = 20%

CURRENT PCV = 16%

DONOR PCV (FROM DONOR OR PIGTAIL) = 36%

BLOOD VOLUME: DOG: 90 ML/KG   CAT: 60 ML/KG

WITH/WITHOUT POST-DONATION I.V. FLUIDS:

WITH: 20%   WITHOUT: 15% (= TOTAL BLOOD VOLUME THAT CAN SAFELY BE REMOVED FROM DONOR)

CALCULATE TOTAL BLOOD VOLUME FROM DONOR:

90 ML/KG X 27.7 KG = 2493 ML TBV

HOW MUCH CAN THE DONOR SAFELY GIVE?

2493 ML X 15% (WITHOUT POST-DONATION FLUIDS) = 373.95 ML

TRANSFUSION VOLUME EQUATION:

(Desired PCV - Current PCV) / (Donor PCV) x (Blood Volume in mL/kg) x (Weight of Recipient in kg)

CALCULATION:

20% - 16% / 36% X 90 ML/KG X 30.3 KG =

4% / 36% X 90 ML/KG X 30.3 KG =

0.04 / 0.36 X 90 ML/KG X 30.3 KG =

0.111 X 90 ML/~~KG~~ X 30.3 ~~KG~~ =

0.111 X 2727 ML (TBV) = 302.697 ML = **303 ML** - TOTAL VOLUME NEEDED BY RECIPIENT FOR A 4% INCREASE IN PCV

CALCULATING BLOOD TRANSFUSION RATES

1. Calculate the Total Volume (in ML) to infuse, divided by the total number of hours in the transfusion
2. Calculate the rate to start slowly and titrate/increase the rate gradually every 15 minutes over the first hour (of 4 hours) of the transfusion
3. Take the inital ML/HR and divide by 4 to determine the first transfusion rate. Divide by 4 because there are 4 15 minute increments in 1 hour
4. At the 15 minute mark if the patient's vitals are stable and no obvious signs for a reaction are seen, then the rate can be doubled for the next 15 minutes
5. Continue to double the rate every 15 minutes for the remainder of the 1st hour, and program the RATE in your pump accordingly every 15 minutes

Example:
250 ML over 4 hours to a 27.7 KG Canine
250 ML / 4 = 62.5 ML/HR
62.5 ML/HR / 4 = 15.625 ML/HR for the 1st 15 minutes
15.625 ML/HR X 2 = 31.25 ML/HR for the next 15 minutes
31.25 ML/HR X 2 = 62.5 ML/HR for the next 15 minutes
62.5 ML/HR X 2 = 125 ML/HR for the next 15 minutes

6. At the 1 hour mark, recalculate infusion rate to administer the remaining volume by calculating the actual TVI by dividing the ML/HR for each 15 minute increment in the first hour by 4 and adding each increment together, or check your pump for the TVI

Example:
15.625 ML/HR / 4 = 3.9 ML
31.25 ML/HR / 4 = 7.8 ML
62.5 ML/HR / 4 = 15.6 ML
125 ML/HR / 4 = 31.25 ML
3.9 ML + 7.8 ML + 15.6 ML + 31.25 ML = 58.5 ML

7. Then take the ML you calculated for the TVI and subtract from your starting volume

Example:
250 ML – 58.5 ML = 191.5 ML REMAINING

8. Then, divide the volume remaining by the hours left to administer the transfusion

Example:
191.5 ML / 3 HR = 63.8 ML/HR – RATE FOR THE NEXT 3 HOURS

9. Then program your pump for 63.8 ML/HR with a VTBI of 191.5 ML and it will be set for the next 3 hours of the transfusion
10. The TVI for the following three hours will be 63.8 ML per hour multiplied by 3 HR which equals 191.4 ML.
11. To calculate ML/KG/HR, take your ML/HR and divide by the patient's weight.

Example:
15.625 ML/HR / 27.7 KG = 0.56 ML/KG/HR – This value is right between 0.5 – 1 ML/KG/HR which is a suggested starting point for transfusions.

Go to http://www.thevettechsguidetoecc.com for a Donor & Recipient Transfusion Calculation Sheet and for a calculated 4 Hour Blood Transfusion Rate Sheet!

MANUAL DRIP (GTT FOR BLOOD TRANSFUSIONS)

ORDER: 60 MLS
TIME: OVER 4 HOURS
DRIP SET: 15 GTT/ML
RATE: X

DRIP SETS = DROPS/MIN

10 DROPS/ML – (ML/HR) / 6 = DROPS/MIN
15 DROPS/ML – (ML/HR) / 4 = DROPS/MIN*
20 DROPS/ML – (ML/HR) / 3 = DROPS/MIN
60 DROPS/ML – (ML/HR) / 1 = DROPS/MIN
* Most frequently carried, double check packaging.

60 ML with 15 DROPS/ML DROP SET over 4 HOURS

DROPS PER MINUTE =
$$\frac{\text{TOTAL VOLUME (ML)}}{\text{TIME (HR)}} \times \frac{\text{DROP FACTOR}}{60 \text{ MIN/HR}}$$

$$\frac{60 \cancel{\text{ML}}}{4 \cancel{\text{HR}}} \times \frac{15 \text{ GTT/}\cancel{\text{ML}}}{60 \text{ MIN/}\cancel{\text{HR}}} = \frac{900 \text{ GTT}}{240 \text{ MIN}} = 3.75 \text{ GTT/MIN}$$

3.75 GTT/MIN = 4 GTT/MIN – ROUND UP TO WHOLE DROP

MANUAL PLATELET COUNT

INSTRUCTIONS:

1. ADD PLATELET COUNT FROM TEN FIELDS OF VIEW.

2. DIVIDE SUM BY 10.

3. MULTIPLY BY 15,000 FOR LOW END.

4. MULTIPLY BY 20,000 FOR HIGH END.

REFERENCE RANGE: >200,000 µL FOR CATS AND DOGS OR 10-24/HPF AT 100X OIL MAGNIFICATION

Transfusion Medicine for the Dog and Cat in the Emergency and Critical Care Setting
Article by Dr. Adam Chung, V.M.D.

Indications
Conditions Requiring Transfusion in the Dog and Cat

Blood Volume in the cat is about 6-8% body weight and about 8-9% body weight in the dog.

Indication for blood transfusion in the dog and cat in the emergency and critical care setting include:

1) Acute blood loss or anemia, although there is no PCV that serves as a trigger for beginning a transfusion, many argue that it should be considered if the PCV drops to 15-17% or sooner based on clinical signs.
2) Coagulopathic conditions such as anticoagulant rodenticides.
3) Coagulation screen prolonged beginning with 70% factor activity loss.
4) Need to consider oxygenation as well; consider when Hgb <7 g/dL.

Transfusion Options

1) **Fresh Whole Blood (FWB)** - RBCs, WBCs, PLTs, albumin, globulin, all clotting factors.
2) **Packed Red Blood Cells (pRBC)** - RBCs +/- some WBCs and inactive PLTs.
3) **Fresh Frozen Plasma (FFP)** - Clotting factors, albumin, globulin.
4) **Frozen Plasma (FP)** - FFP that has been stored for 1-5 years, deficient in factor V, VIII, vWF.
5) **Platelet rich plasma** - PLT, WBCs; can be spun again to obtain platelet concentrate.
6) **Cryo-poor plasma** - Contains albumin, globulins, and coagulation factors 2, 7, 9, 10.
7) **Cryoprecipitate** - Contains coagulation factor 8 and vWF, along with XIII and fibrinogen.

What to Tranfuse

1) **Replace what is lost:**
   a) Ex: A euvolemic patient can experience hemolysis and only need red blood cells; thus, pRBCs would be more appropriate than FWB.
2) **Plasma:**
   a) These transfusions are controversial, particularly for issues such as DIC and hypoalbuminemia; some blood banks will withhold plasma if the intended use is for these conditions.
   b) Accepted use is for patients that are hemorrhaging and have exhausted their clotting factors.
   c) Patients with deficiency in stable clotting factors and PT/aPTT are prolonged.
3) **Platelets:**
   a) Used when patients are experiencing life-threatening hemorrhage secondary to platelet disorders.
   b) Not commonly used for aclinical forms of thrombocytopenia.

Testing Prior to Transfusions
Blood Typing and Crossmatching

1) **Blood type** - The safest recommendation is to blood type before giving any blood product.
   a) There are greater than 12 blood types in dogs; most common type that will cause a reaction is DEA 1.
   b) In crisis situations- whether the owner cannot afford blood typing, time is of the essence, or there is a limitation on blood products, a dog can receive DEA 1 positive or negative blood **as long as they do not have a prior history of receiving a transfusion.**
      i) Note: Giving DEA 1 blood to a patient that does not have DEA 1 blood will lead to antibody production, decrease the lifespan of the RBCs, and will make a future transfusion reaction much more likely.
      ii) Thus, it is ideal to only give DEA 1 negative blood if type unknown

Transfusion Medicine for the Dog and Cat in the Emergency and Critical Care Setting
Article by Dr. Adam Chung, V.M.D.

c) Cats are commonly tested as A, B, or AB and are born with antibodies against other blood types.
   i) Thus, MUST blood type **ALL** cats prior to a transfusion.
d) Note: Cats do not have antibodies against canine blood and therefore xenotransfusion has been described in life threatening circumstances.
   i) This can only be done **once** in a cat's lifetime, as they will develop antibodies.

2) **Crossmatch** - This is also recommended prior to transfusing red blood cell products.
   a) Major: Donor cells and recipient plasma are mixed and monitored for agglutination, which represents hemolysis and an incompatibility.
      i) Recommended in ideally all patients and especially those that have received a transfusion in the past, more than 5 days ago.
   b) Minor: Donor plasma with recipient cells.

Calculating the Volume to Tranfuse

Red blood cells
1) The previous school of thought of 1mL/kg of blood per desired % increase in PCV has shifted to the following:
   a) Whole blood preparations: 2mL/kg body weight will increase the PCV by 1%.
   b) pRBC preparations: 1.5mL/kg body weight will increase the PCV by 1%.
2) A common goal is a 10% increase in PCV, although a starting dose of 6-10mL/kg is practical.
3) During massive transfusion, a 1:1 ratio of pRBCs and plasma is recommended to avoid dilutional coagulopathy.

Plasma
1) A typical starting dose for a plasma transfusion is 10-20mL/kg body weight.
2) Monitoring clotting parameters and evidence of continued bleeding recommended to determine if further transfusions are necessary.
3) Some cite that upwards of 40mL/kg of plasma is needed to increase the patient's albumin by 1g/dL.

Pre-medicating

1) Premedicating with diphenhydramine and/or steroids are not required. Studies have shown that these can be effective in reducing mild hypersensitivity reactions (i.e. facial swelling, pruritus, etc.), but does not diminish the risk of anaphylaxis.

Beginning the Transfusion

1) RBC products <u>should not be warmed</u> unless large volumes are given to a small patient, the patient is hypothermic, or a large volume is needed.
2) Warming can degenerate coagulation factors or allow bacteria to grow.
3) Plasma products should be thawed at room temperature.

Running the Transfusion

1) A 160-260 micron gravity drip filter is optimal for red blood cell survival.
2) If fluid support is needed during a transfusion, the fluid of choice can be run through a **separate** catheter, or 0.9% NaCl can be run through the same catheter via Y-piece adapter.
   a) Remember to take product volume into account in regards to fluid replacement.
3) If mild-moderate clinical signs are seen in the patient, the transfusion can be given over a 4-hour period; a longer duration can predispose the unit to bacterial proliferation.
   a) If large volumes are required, keep additional units cool until they are needed.
   b) Begin the transfusion slowly (0.5-1mL/kg/hr) while monitoring temperature, pulse,

Transfusion Medicine for the Dog and Cat in the Emergency and Critical Care Setting   *Article by Dr. Adam Chung, V.M.D.*

respiratory rate, MM, and CRT q10-15 min.

c) If tolerating the transfusion well after the first 30 minutes, can double the rate for the next 30 minutes, followed by an increase to a rate that completes the transfusion within 2-4 hours, while monitoring vitals and reactions every hour.

4) For severe/life threatening cases, blood can be bolused immediately or administered over 1-2 hours.

Peri-Transfusion Monitoring

1) Record pre-transfusion vital parameters and check every 15 minutes for the first hour and then every 30 minutes to one hour if the transfusion is well tolerated.
2) The patient's heart rate and respiratory rate are expected to decrease as the patient responds and hypovolemia and hypoxia are addressed; if these increases during this time period, this could be a sign of a transfusion reaction.
3) Febrile non-hemolytic conditions can arise throughout the transfusion.
   a) This is thought to be secondary to antibodies responding to antigens on the donor's WBCs.

Transfusion Reactions

1) If there is a concern for a mild transfusion reaction, reduce the rate by 25-50% and track changes in the vital parameters.
2) If a fever is seen in conjunction with cardiovascular changes, the transfusion may need to be discontinued.
3) Acute hemolysis occurs when the recipient's antibodies bind to the donor's RBC surface antigens.
   a) This is typically seen within the first hour of a transfusion.
   b) Common signs include fever, tachypnea, shock, vomiting, and possibly death.
4) If there is any concern for hemolysis, check for slide agglutination or hematocrit tube for evidence of pink serum; the transfusion will need to be stopped at this time and supportive care instituted- IV fluids, anti-emetics, oxygen supplementation, etc.
   a) Note: This will be difficult to assess with IMHA patients.
5) Anaphylaxis is uncommon, but the transfusion should be stopped and epinephrine administered.
6) Transfusion-Related Acute Lung Injury (TRALI)- Acute respiratory distress resembling an ARDS response.
   a) This results in protein leakage and infiltration of inflammatory cells into the lung parenchyma, leading to respiratory distress and hypoxemia.
   b) This can occur within 6 hours of a transfusion and may require O2 supplementation or mechanical ventilation.
      i) Be sure to rule out cardiac issues or volume overload.

Repeat Transfusions

1) Based on clinical improvement in combination with laboratory data.
   a) PCV should be rechecked shortly after the transfusion has finished.
   b) Evaluate the plasma for icterus or signs of hemolysis.
2) Unused blood products can be refrigerated and used within 24 hours.

References

Davidow, Beth. Transfusion Medicine in Small Animals. Veterinary Clinics: Small Animal Practice; 2013; 43.4: 735-756

Giger, U. Transfusion medicine. In: Silverstein DC, Hopper K, eds. Small Animal Critical Care Medicine. St. Louis: Elsevier Saunders; 2009:281-286

Hohenhaus, A.E. Blood Banking and Transfusion Medicine. In: Ettinger SJ, Feldman EC, eds. *Textbook of Veterinary Internal Medicine* (5th ed., Vol 1) St.

CHAPTER 15:
ANESTHESIA SHEET

Anesthetic Monitoring Sheet

<table>
<tr><td>Patient Label Here</td></tr>
</table>

ASA Classification: **Date/Time:** _____

I II III IV V   **Doctor:** _____

IVC Size: ___ **GA** ___ **Loc** **Anesthetist:** _____

IVC Size: ___ **GA** ___ **Loc** **Procedure(s):** _____

Patient History/Clinical Findings:

_____

_____

_____

Local Block: _____

Location: _____

ETT: _____ **MM**   **Patient Weight:** _____ kg   **BCS:** ___ /9

Code Status: CPR DNR   **Body Position:** _____   **Flow-By:** Y N

Circuit: Rebreather Non-rebreather **Surgical IV Fluids & Rate:** _____ mL/hr

Typical Sx Rate K9: 5-10mL/kg/hr; Feline: 3mL/kg/hr

Antibiotics: Cefazolin 100mg/mL 22mg/kg IV = _____ mL

Pre-op _____ AM PM *Intra-op* q90m _____ AM PM _____ AM PM *Post-op* _____ AM PM

Unasyn 30mg/mL 30-50mg/kg IV = _____ mL

Pre-op _____ AM PM *Intra-op* q90m _____ AM PM _____ AM PM *Post-op* _____ AM PM

Baytril 22.7mg/mL 5-10mg/kg IV = _____ mL SID

Pre-op Vitals & Bloodwork

Temp	HR	RR	MM/CRT	BP	PCV	TS	BG	Lactate	BUN	CREA	____

Pre-Med's
Drug	Order	mL	Route	Time
____	_____	__	_____	____
____	_____	__	_____	____
____	_____	__	_____	____

Induction
Drug	Order	mL	Route	Time
____	_____	__	_____	____
____	_____	__	_____	____

CRI Loading Doses
Drug	Order	T.V.	Route	Time
____	_____	____	_____	____
____	_____	____	_____	____
____	_____	____	_____	____

CRI Drugs & Doses
Drug	Order	Rate	T.V.	Time
____	_____	____	____	____
____	_____	____	____	____
____	_____	____	____	____

Anesthesia Machine Checklist:

Reservoir Bag Size: _____ /L

10-20mL x (BW$_{kg}$) x 6, then convert from mL to L

Leak Tests: *Surgery Prep:* **PASS FAIL**
  Surgery: **PASS FAIL**

Eyes Lubed ☐

O2 Flow Rate Checklist:

Rebreathing: 25-50mL/kg/min = _____ L/min

Not less than 500mL/min (0.5L/min) in any patient

Non-rebreathing: 200-300mL/kg/min = _____ L/min

Not less than 500mL/min (0.5L/min) in any patient (Circle system)

Pop Off Valve Re-Opened: Surgery Prep ☐ Surgery ☐

Isoflurane Checklist:

Isoflurane filled to line: *Surgery Prep* ☐
  Surgery ☐

Induction: ___ % **Maintenance:** ___ %

Anesthesia Start Time: _____ AM PM

Anesthesia End Time: _____ AM PM

Procedure 1 Start Time: _____ AM PM

Procedure 1 End Time: _____ AM PM

Intubation Time: _____ AM PM

Extubation Time: _____ AM PM

Procedure 2 Start Time: _____ AM PM

Procedure 2 End Time: _____ AM PM

Post-Op Orders: _____

_____

_____

Patient Weight: _____ kg

Surgical Maintenance Fluids
K9: 60mL/kg/day; Feline: 40mL/kg/day = 1xM
Typical Sx Rate K9: 5-10mL/kg/hr; Feline: 3mL/kg/hr

Fluid Type: _____

Pre-Op Maintenance IV Fluids: _____ mL/hr

Sx Rate: _____ mL/hr *(Sx Rate = 3-10mL/kg/hr)*

Post-Op Maintenance IV Fluids: _____ mL/hr

Colloid Bolus Information
6% HES: K9: ¼ dose = 5mL/kg/day; Feline: ¼ dose = 2.5mL/kg/day
6% HES: K9: Total Dose = 20mL/kg/day; Feline: Total Dose = 10mL/kg/day
First 10-20mL SLOW

Pre-Op Colloid Bolus: _____ = RATE _____ = VTBI

_____ = RATE _____ = VTBI

Intra-Op Colloid Bolus: _____ = RATE _____ = VTBI

Post-Op Colloid Bolus: _____ = RATE _____ = VTBI

_____ = RATE _____ = VTBI

Crystalloid Bolus Information
K9 ¼ Shock Bolus Aliquot: 20mL/kg
Feline ¼ Shock Bolus Aliquot: 5mL/kg

Fluid Type: _____

Pre-Op Crystalloid Bolus: _____ = RATE _____ = VTBI

_____ = RATE _____ = VTBI

Intra-Op Crystalloid Bolus: _____ = RATE _____ = VTBI

_____ = RATE _____ = VTBI

Post-op Crystalloid Bolus: _____ = RATE _____ = VTBI

_____ = RATE _____ = VTBI

CAUTION BOLUSING IN CARDIAC AND RENAL IMPAIRED PATIENTS

Colloid Maintenance Information
6% HES: K9: 20mL/kg/day; Feline: 10mL/kg/day
Run at 1mL/kg/hr

Maintenance Rate: _____ mL/hr

Maintenance Total Volume: _____ mL

Total Volume of Fluids Administered during Procedure(s): _____ mL

Anesthetic Emergency Drug Information

DRUGS	MG	ML	ROUTE	TIME GIVEN	NOTES
Atropine 0.4mg/mL **0.02-0.04mg/kg IV**					
Glycopyrrolate 0.2mg/mL **0.005-0.011mg/kg IV**					
Naloxone 0.4mg/mL **0.02mg/kg IV** *Dilute 1:10 and adm. over 1 min*					
Flumazenil 0.1mg/mL **0.01mg/kg IV**					
Lidocaine 20mg/mL **Feline: 0.2-0.7mg/kg** 1mg/kg max **K9: 2-4mg/kg IV**					
Epi Low 1mg/mL **0.01mg/kg IV**					
Epi High 1mg/mL **0.1mg/kg IV**					
Insulin (Humulin-R) **0.25-0.5U/kg IV**					
Dextrose 50% **1mL/kg IV** *Dilute at least 1:4*					
Calcium Gluconate 10% **0.5-1.5mL/kg IV** *Slowly over 5-10 mins (ECG required)*					
_____ _____ mg/mL					

Time	00 Hr	05	10	15	20	25	30	35	40	45	50	55	00 Hr	05	10	15	20	25	30	35	40	45	50	55
HR																								
SpO2																								
EtCO2																								
RR																								
Temp																								
Sys BP																								
Dia BP																								
MAP BP																								
ISO																								
O2																								
ECG																								
IVF Rate																								
CRI Rate																								
ABX																								
Notes																								

Emergency CRI's

Dobutamine 12.5mg/mL: *Positive Inotrope*; *No L.D.*; *CRI Dosing Range: K9: 0.3mg/kg/hr - 1.2mg/kg/hr = 5 - 20mcg/kg/min; Feline: 0.15 - 0.9mg/kg/hr = 2.5 - 15mcg/kg/min;* **Dilute 1.5mL Dobutamine in 60mL of 0.9% NaCl, giving a dilution of 300mcg/mL. Start at 1mL/kg/hr which is 5mcg/kg/min. Increase up to 4mL/kg/hr IV.**

Dopamine 40mg/mL: *Positive Inotrope; Vasopressor; No L.D.; CRI Dosing Range: K9 & Feline: 0.12 - 1.2mg/kg/hr = 2 - 20mcg/kg/min;* **Dilute 0.3mL Dopamine in 60mL of 0.9% NaCl, giving a dilution of 0.2mg/mL = 200mcg/mL. Start at 0.6mL/kg/hr = 2mcg/kg/min. Run @ 1 - 2mL/kg/hr for moderate hypotension; for severe hypotension 3 - 4 mL/kg/hr. Increase up to 6mL/kg/hr if necessary.** *Preferred for cats, studies unsure if cat's have the receptors for Dobutamine despite availability of dosing information above.*

Lidocaine 2% / 20mg/mL: *Anti-Arrhythmic; L.D.: K9: 2mg/kg; Feline: 0.2-0.7mg/kg; CRI Dosing Range: K9: 1.5 - 4.8mg/kg/hr = 25 - 80mcg/kg/min; Feline: 0.6 - 1.2mg/kg/hr = 10 - 20mcg/kg/min;* **K9: Start CRI @ 1.5mg/kg/hr = 25mcg/kg/min IV. Increase up to 4.8mg/kg/hr = 80mcg/kg/min. Feline: Start CRI @ 0.6mg/kg/hr = 10mcg/kg/min IV. Increase up to 1.2mg/kg/hr = 20mcg/kg/min.** *No need to dilute if only drug on syringe pump. To get rate, divide mg/hr by concentration = mL/hr.*

Norepinephrine 1mg/mL: *Vasopressor;* <u>*Must be diluted in 0.9% NaCl. TITRATE TO EFFECT.*</u> *No L.D.; CRI Dosing Range: K9 & Feline: 0.006 - 0.12mg/kg/hr = 0.1 - 2mcg/kg/min (0.4mcg/kg/min median effective dose). Onset of action 1 – 2 minutes, titrate dosage up in increments of 3 minutes until desired effect achieved. Continually monitor BP, goal MAP = >65mmHg, Continuous ECG, and UOP monitoring REQUIRED.* **Dilute 1.45mL of Norepi in 60mL 0.9% NaCl, giving a dilution of 24mcg/mL. Start CRI at 0.25mL/kg/hr. Increase up to 5mL/kg/hr.**

Calculations

CRI Monitoring Record

Drug	Order	Total Volume (Drug : Diluent) in mL	Rate	Notes
Dobutamine 12.5mg/mL				
Dopamine 40mg/mL				
Lidocaine 20mg/mL				
Norepinephrine 1mg/mL				

Post-op Vitals & Bloodwork

Temp	HR	RR	MM/CRT	BP	PCV	TS	BG	Lactate	BUN	CREA	____

Anesthetic Notes

CHAPTER 16:
TIPS & TRICKS FROM VETERINARY PROFESSIONALS

Tips and Tricks
from Veterinary Professionals

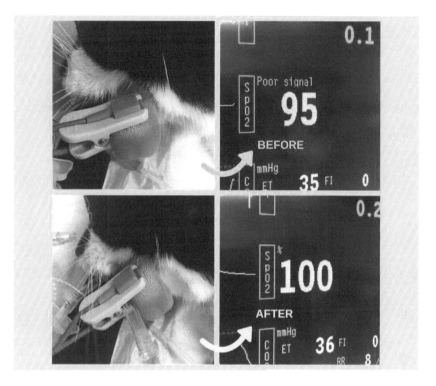

Tip: SpO2 Machine Hack

"Here is my snazzy hack for making the pulse oximeter work on tiny tongues when the probe itself compresses the capillary bed so much it has nothing to read! I wedge it open with a needle cap. (Some people use a swab too but it may not always be able to read through that.) You can actually see how tight the probe is in the first picture as the tongue is even a little bit blue where it is cutting off the perfusion! Real world tips from a real world VN!"

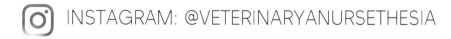 INSTAGRAM: @VETERINARYANURSETHESIA

Tip: Don't underestimate the value of the patient's history and physical examination

"One of the best tips I can give to anyone treating a patient that has presented for an emergency is to not ignore the history and physical exam of the animal. It can be easy to focus on the presenting complaint and start a comprehensive targeted diagnostic work up. Rather than that, stabilizing the patient and acquiring a thorough history can give you an important piece of the presenting puzzle. A full physical exam will not only give you relevant information related to the underlying cause of the patient's problem. It also gives you a baseline status of the animal for monitoring purposes and can identify other problems to add to your problem list. It is vital to treat every pet as a new patient and gain as much of the clinical picture as possible, particularly with history taking and a physical examination."

 INSTAGRAM: @DOGTORBIANCA

Tip: Estimating a patient's weight in an emergency

The Beagle Rule: "Use this as a guide to estimate weight for unstable or emergent patients. To visualize the patient's weight, think of a lean, young, 22lb. Beagle and the size that this would be. (22 lb = 10 kg) How many Beagles would it take to be this animal in front of you? Let's say it's really a 19 kg canine, looking at him and eyeballing it, it would take about 2 Beagles to make up this patient so that means 10 kg per Beagle = 20 kg patient"

 INSTAGRAM: @THEVETTECHSGUIDETOECC

CHAPTER 17: CAPNOGRAPHY

CAPNOGRAPHY

Sometimes things are just better shown -or drawn- than just explained. This book was derived from two handwritten books and I wanted you to see some of that in this book, and I wanted to pay some homage to them, so here is my section on CAPNOGRAPHY, my absolute favorite vital monitoring parameter.

Capnography measures end-tidal CO2 (EtCO2), which is the amount of CO_2 present in exhaled air. It also displays a waveform that represents air movement during the respiratory cycle. EtCO2 is normally 35-45 mmHg and the waveform is normally rectangular in shape. The waveform provides breath-to-breath feedback about the patient's respiratory rate, ventilation, perfusion/cardiac output, proper/improper intubation, efficacy of chest compressions, and cellular metabolism. During anesthesia, we want our patients to be between 35-45. During CPR 15-25 tells us there is perfusion, but just 10 is what we should aim for. A lot of techs haven't been taught about EtCO2 capnograms, so here is some great material from my handwritten books and from a conference I attended!

Capnography tells us:	ABNORMAL
-Ventilation -Cardiac Output -Intubation -Chest Compressions -Cellular Metabolism	<15 DANGEROUS <35 HYPOCAPNIA >45 HYPERCAPNIA >60 DANGEROUS
15-25 mmHg is PERFUSION 35-45 mmHg is NORMAL	BEWARE of an >60 EtCO2, this itself can become an anesthetic and will deepen your patient further than they already are.

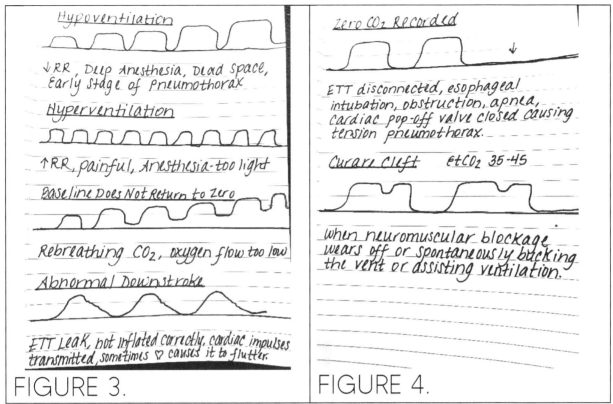

FIGURES 3, 4. Lake, K., (2019).

**In Figure 3, spontaneous bucking can also be seen as an Abnormal Downstroke waveform.

**In Figure 4, zero CO2 recorded can also be interpreted as the patient is no longer breathing/cardiopulmonary arrest and CPR should begin if this is the case.

Normal Capnogram

The normal capnogram is a waveform which represents the varying CO_2 level throughout the breath cycle.

Waveform Characteristics:

A-B: Baseline **D:** End-Tidal Concentration
B-C: Expiratory Upstroke **D-E:** Inspiration
C-D: Expiratory Plateau

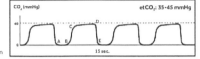

Rebreathing CO₂

Other Possible Causes:

- Faulty expiratory valve
- Inadequate inspiratory flow
- Partial rebreathing
- Insufficient expiratory time

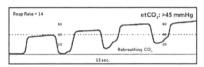

Bronchospasm/Asthma

Other Possible Causes:

- Bronchospasm/COPD
- Obstruction in the expiratory limb of the breathing circuit
- Presence of a foreign body in the upper airway
- Partially kinked or occluded artificial airway

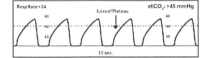

Curare Cleft

Other Possible Causes:

- Patient is mechanically ventilated
- Depth of cleft is proportional to degree of muscle relaxants

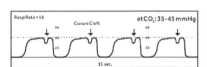

*Increasing etCO₂ (Hypoventilation)

Other Possible Causes:

- Decrease in respiratory rate
- Decrease in tidal volume
- Increase in metabolic rate
- Rapid rise in body temperature (malignant hyperthermia)

Cardiac Arrest

Other Possible Causes:

- Decreased or absent cardiac output
- Decreased or absent pulmonary blood flow
- Sudden decrease in CO_2 values

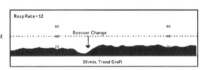

*Decreasing etCO₂ (Hyperventilation)

Other Possible Causes:

- Increase in respiratory rate
- Increase in tidal volume
- Metabolic acidosis
- Fall in body temperature

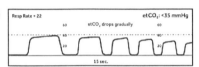

Return of Spontaneous Circulation

Other Possible Causes:

- Increase in cardiac output
- Increase in pulmonary blood flow
- Gradual increase in CO_2 production

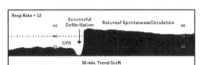

*Assumes adequate circulation and alveolar gas exchange

Medtronic
Further Together

FIGURE 5.

FIGURE 5. MEDTRONIC, (2019).

CHAPTER 18:
EMERGENCY MEDICINE AND HOW TO THRIVE IN AN UNKNOWN ENVIRONMENT

Emergency Medicine and How to Thrive in an Unknown Environment
Article by Dr. Bianca Ferlisi D.V.M.

The emergency room is inevitably a high stress area in an animal hospital. It can be a daunting place, particularly for those who are unfamiliar with it. This includes students, doctors, and technicians, with varying levels of experience. What is it about emergency medicine that is so intimidating? There are many key factors that must be considered when evaluating this question.

Usually, patients presenting to emergency services are in critical condition and require immediate intervention. Though a presenting problem can sometimes be easily identified, there is often a large, unknown aspect of what is wrong with the patient that must be determined. This requires a financial conversation with an owner followed by a diagnostic work up once the patient is stabilized. Unfortunately, the degree of variation in emergency cases does not allow for a simple flow chart to follow when handling cases. Some may be more complicated than others from a medical standpoint, while others may be straightforward medicine on an animal with difficult owners. Even so, there are principles that may be implemented in each case, especially for a person who is not well-versed in emergency medicine, to maximize the probability of success.

Try to Know What You Do Not Know

It can be difficult for many people to acknowledge when they do not know something. It seems like a simple notion, but having self-awareness and recognizing when you do not know an answer is an imperative skill, especially in emergency medicine. As a new graduate, it may be defeating to not know every test that should be run, every normal reference range, how to perform every clinical skill, and every differential diagnosis. The list of what one must know in veterinary medicine is endless, and expecting yourself to know everything, especially as someone just entering the field of emergency medicine, is unrealistic. Rather, it is more productive to study, actively learn, and be aware when you do not know an answer. It is more useful to have knowledge of appropriate resources to find relevant information as opposed to formulating an incorrect response for the sake of pride. This will not only allow for optimal patient care, but it will also exemplify your dependability in the emergency setting. Your colleagues will have confidence that you are providing accurate information, rather than something you came up with in place of not having an answer. This confidence allows for a foundation of trust and teamwork to be built amongst the doctors and technicians – something that is imperative in an emergency setting.

The Three Right's: Right Dose, Right Route, Right Patient

Checking your medications and treatments before administering them is a crucial habit not only in emergency practice but in veterinary medicine as a whole. A simple check of correct dose, route, and animal can provide confidence that your patient is receiving the appropriate therapy. There are times when emergency rooms can be chaotic, when you are fatigued from a long shift, or when you are not focused on the task at hand. These are all examples of scenarios that can lead to a potentially fatal error with medication administration. Whether you have never before given that specific medication, or if you are comfortable with it and have used it numerous times, you should always double check prior to administration. It is inevitable that mistakes will be made throughout your career, especially as a new graduate. Reducing the amount of avoidable errors by double checking is a way to minimize this.

Emergency Medicine and How to Thrive in an Unknown Environment
Article by Dr. Bianca Ferlisi D.V.M.

Great Communication and Efficiency are Key

In critical settings, it is essential to be honest with your fellow doctors and technicians, as well as pet owners. Communication is vital in any animal hospital, but it is especially crucial in critical cases where efficiency is key. An owner bringing their pet to an emergency practice will likely be worried and require some form of reassurance. It is your duty as the person that will be caring for the animal to be honest about cost of care, prognosis, and plans moving forward. Having a printed estimate that is reviewed and signed by an owner can be a clear explanation of the financial aspect of an emergency visit. Explaining why each test is being run and what your thoughts are regarding the case builds rapport with clients. Discuss the prognosis, and through helping a client set realistic goals and limits, try to then discuss any otherwise unexpected scenarios that may arise during intervention. Though emergency medicine is unpredictable, taking as much of the unknown out of the situation as possible can provide necessary comfort for the client.

In addition to communicating openly with clients, it is essential to communicate with fellow technicians and doctors. Whether it be running a code, planning treatment protocols or discussing a case. Being on the same page allows for efficiency and maximum productivity with limited discrepancies. As a new person in an emergency setting, asking for help and seeking information regarding procedures, cases and treatment plans is an excellent method of learning and becoming more comfortable with the realm of emergency medicine. It also informs those around you of your level of experience, so you are not expected to have skills or knowledge that you may not have yet. Consciously practicing communication skills as a new technician or doctor in an emergency setting will lead to development of good communication habits that over time, become natural and routine.

Empathy – Feeling With, Not For, People

One of the most important skills a veterinarian or technician can master is the ability to empathize. One must look at the emergency appointment not as a 'business as usual' type of visit. Instead, perceive it from the pet owner's point of view - an unplanned trip to the veterinarian with associated costs, a beloved pet in distress, and all the worry that surrounds that. Clients may handle this stress in a variety of ways including tears, anger, confusion, or irritation. Understanding the root of these feelings and being able to empathize with the owner builds a positive relationship. As mentioned before, it is essential that the details of the case be communicated to the pet owner. Unfortunately, there are times that there are no answers to relay. It could be that diagnostic test results are pending, or a new plan has yet to be formed. It is especially important at those times to practice empathy with your clients. There are many strategies that you can implement to display empathy. Actively listening, recognizing your client's emotions, and staying out of judgement are a few key aspects of empathy. The overall goal should be to put yourself in a place of understanding how your client is feeling and where they are coming from.

Practice Self Care

The unfortunate reality of emergency medicine is that many patients pass away despite the emergency team's best efforts. In addition, many emergency shifts are long and encompass odd hours of the day. The inevitable fatigue and exposure to death and suffering can take a toll on a person. Finding hobbies outside of veterinary medicine and taking time to care for yourself is the key to a healthy veterinary career. Finding moments to self-reflect and

Emergency Medicine and How to Thrive in an Unknown Environment *Article by Dr. Bianca Ferlisi D.V.M.*

evaluate your mental state are necessary. Learning to define yourself outside of veterinary medicine and giving yourself time to recharge will improve your well-being, not only during your emergency shifts, but in your life as a whole.

Conclusion

Though entering an emergency setting for the first time can be overwhelming, practicing and mastering the skills above can optimize growth and minimize obstacles that one will inevitably be faced with when being involved in emergency medicine. With the support of a cohesive team, and self-awareness of the development of these skills, emergency medicine can be rewarding and fulfilling, instead of intimidating.

CHAPTER 19:
CITATIONS

CITATIONS

FIGURES

FIGURE 1
RapidVet-H Major Crossmatch Kit Procedure Card. Rapidvet.com https://www.rapidvet.com/pdf/2013_x_major_card.pdf [Accessed 05 Jan. 2023.]

FIGURE 2
RapidVet-H Crossmatch Photo Identifier. RapidVet.com. (n.d.). Retrieved February 13, 2023, from http://www.rapidvet.com/pdf/CM-PhotoID.12-17_1pg.pdf

FIGURES 3, 4
Lake K. *The Veterinary Technician's Guide to Emergency and Critical Care*. 1st ed. Alexandria, VA: Writer's Republic.

FIGURE 5
Normal and abnormal capnography waveforms infographic - CapnoAcademy. CapnoAcademy. https://www.capnoacademy.com/2018/10/03/normal-and-abnormal-capnography-waveforms-infographic/. Published 2019. [Accessed 19 Dec. 2019.]

TABLES

TABLE 1
Muir WW, DiBartola SP. Fluid therapy. In: Kirk RW, ed. *Current Veterinary Therapy VIII*. Philadelphia: WB Saunders; 1983:33.

CITATIONS CONTINUED

TABLE 2
Tabor, B. (2022, June 20). *Shock: An overview*. Today's Veterinary Nurse. Retrieved February 13, 2023, from https://todaysveterinarynurse.com/emergency-medicine-critical-care/shock-an-overview/

TABLE 3
Silverstein, D., & Proulx, A. (2022, February 18). *Resuscitative fluid therapy for circulatory shock*. Today's Veterinary Practice. Retrieved February 13, 2023, from https://todaysveterinarypractice.com/emergency-medicine-critical-care/resuscitative-fluid-therapy-for-circulatory-shock/

TABLE 4
Hare, W., Post, L. and Oehme, F. (n.d.). *A Review of Veterinary Antidotes*. [online] American Board of Veterinary Toxicology. Available at: https://www.abvt.org/public/docs/reviewofveterinaryantidotes.pdf [Accessed 4 Sep. 2019].

TABLE 5
Fletcher, D. J., Boller, M., Brainard, B. M., Haskins, S. C., Hopper, K., McMichael, M. A., Rozanski, E. A., Rush, J. E., Smarick, S. D., American College of Veterinary Medicine, & Veterinary Emergency and Critical Care Society (2012). RECOVER evidence and knowledge gap analysis on veterinary CPR. Part 7: Clinical guidelines. *Journal of veterinary emergency and critical care (San Antonio, Tex. : 2001), 22 Suppl 1*, S102–S131. https://doi.org/10.1111/j.1476-4431.2012.00757.x

CITATIONS CONTINUED

TABLE 6

Plumbsveterinarydrugs.com. (2019). *Plumb's Veterinary Drugs*. [online] Available at: https://www.plumbsveterinarydrugs.com [Accessed 17 Dec. 2019].

IMAGES

IMAGE #1

Boag, A. (2015). *Vascular Compartments Image*. Veterinary Information Network. Retrieved 2023, from https://www.vin.com/AppUtil/Image/handler.ashx?imgid=3418401&w=&h=.

Snake Bite Envenomation Protocol Clinical Pathology Images

A resource for veterinary clinical pathology. eClinpath. (2021, November 3). Retrieved February 13, 2023, from https://eclinpath.com/

Snake Bite Envenomation Protocol Alvedia Quick Test Blood Typing Images

Alvedia.com. Alvedia. (n.d.). Retrieved February 13, 2023, from https://www.alvedia.com/

ARTICLES REFERENCED

Boag, A. (2015). *Shock Assessment and Treatment (Basic) – WSAVA 2015 Congress - VIN*. Powered By VIN. https://www.vin.com/apputil/content/defaultadv1.aspx?pId=14365&catId=736 80&id=7259218.

CITATIONS CONTINUED

Brown DE, Meyer DJ, Wingfield WE, Walton RM. Echinocytosis associated with rattlesnake envenomation in dogs. Vet Pathol. 1994 Nov;31(6):654-7. doi: 10.1177/030098589403100604. PMID: 7863580.

Lyons, B. M., & Waddell, L. S. (2019, August 22). Fluid Therapy in Hospitalized Patients, Part 1: Patient Assessment and Fluid Choices. Retrieved from https://todaysveterinarypractice.com/fluid-therapy-part-1fluid-therapy-hospitalized-patients-patient-assessment-fluid-choices/

Najman, L., & Seshadri, R. (2007, March). *Rattlesnake Envenomation*. Vetfolio. Retrieved February 13, 2023, from https://www.vetfolio.com/learn/article/rattlesnake-envenomation

Péterfi, O., Boda, F., Szabó, Z., Ferencz, E., & Bába, L. (2019). Hypotensive Snake Venom Components-A Mini-Review. *Molecules (Basel, Switzerland), 24*(15), 2778. https://doi.org/10.3390/molecules24152778

Snakebite: Facing the Challenges - WSAVA2013 - VIN . (2023). Retrieved 5 January 2023, from https://www.vin.com/apputil/content/defaultadv1.aspx?pId=11372&meta=generic&catId=35323&id=5709822&ind=158&objTypeID=17

Walton RM, Brown DE, Hamar DW, et al: Mechanisms of echinocytosis induced by *Crotalus atrox* venom. *Vet Pathol* 34:442-449, 1997.

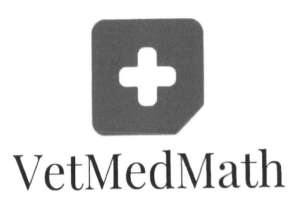

Thank You

WRITER'S REPUBLIC

DR. ADAM CHUNG, VMD

DR. BIANCA FERLISI, DVM

BRIAN GOLEMAN, RVT

ASHLEY JOYCE, RVT

ANNE LINDSAY, LVT, CVPP, CCRP, CCMT, FFCP, OACM, VTS CLINICAL PRACTICE (CANINE/FELINE)

MY VETERINARY COMMUNITY

MY FAMILY AND FRIENDS

THANK YOU ALL FOR YOUR SUPPORT

LEGAL

Veterinary medicine is constantly in a state of flux and its information is continually growing daily. The information contained in this book is up-to-date as of March 2023. Information will continue to be revised in future editions to stay current with trends in Veterinary Medicine. This book is foundational in nature and the skills discussed in this book will be built upon in future books. The Veterinary field utilizes drugs in a variety of ways, therefore drug concentrations may be different in your hospital, so please double check the bottle you are working with. The drug concentrations presented are the most commonly used in Emergency Veterinary Medicine, but that's not to say they are the only concentrations used. The author of this book is not liable for any errors made due to its consultation. All drug dosages and treatments should be double checked by a Licensed Veterinary Technician and a Doctor of Veterinary Medicine before providing them to a patient.

CPSIA information can be obtained
at www.ICGtesting.com
Printed in the USA
LVHW071047270723
753638LV00002B/3